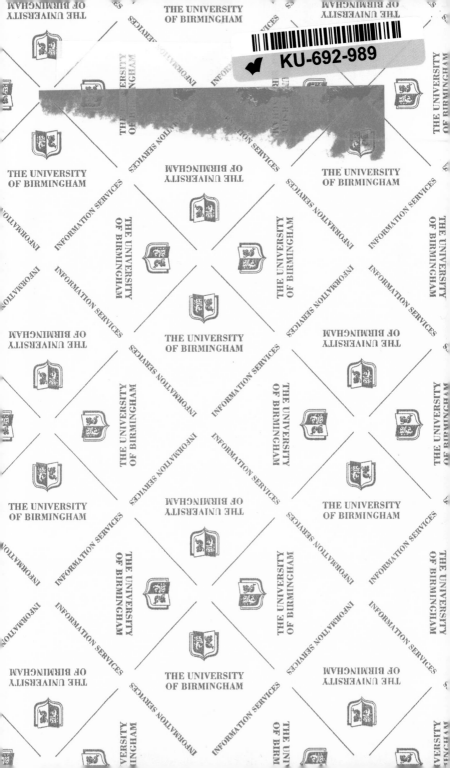

Michael W. DeGregorio
and Valerie J. Wiebe

Tamoxifen and Breast Cancer

Yale University Press

New Haven and London

Designed by Nancy Ovedovitz. Set in New Baskerville type by The Composing Room of Michigan, Inc., Grand Rapids, Michigan. Printed in the United States of America by Vail-Ballou Press, Binghamton, New York.

Library of Congress Cataloging-in-Publication Data

DeGregorio, Michael W., 1955–
Tamoxifen and breast cancer / Michael W. DeGregorio and Valerie J. Wiebe.
    p. cm.
  Includes bibliographical references and index.
  ISBN 0-300-05907-8 (cloth). — ISBN 0-300-05992-2 (pbk).
  1. Tamoxifen. 2. Breast—Cancer—Chemoprevention. I. Wiebe, Valerie J., 1958–   . II. Title.
RC280.B8D39   1994
616.99′44905—dc20   93-43148
                       CIP

A catalogue record for this book is available from the British Library.

The paper in this book meets the guidelines for permanence and durability of the Committee on Production Guidelines for Book Longevity of the Council on Library Resources.

10   9   8   7   6   5   4   3   2   1

Contents

Preface

Approximately one woman in nine will develop breast cancer in her lifetime. The most common form of cancer found in women, breast cancer is devastating socially, psychologically, and physically in ways that too often are considered secondary to the disease process itself. The diagnosis is frightening, but so are the choices that must be made after diagnosis. And little clear-cut information is available on what form of treatment is best for specific stages or types of breast cancer.

Decisions are needed not only on the type of surgery, if any, to be performed but also on the type of therapy that should follow. Radiation, chemotherapy, and hormonal therapy are all options to be considered. Radiation therapy has proved itself in specific patients and is accepted by most clinicians, but the value of many drug therapies in breast cancer is ambiguous. Although these treatments are effective for some patients, other women derive less benefit from the same drugs.

The use of tamoxifen and other hormonal agents is even more debatable. Tamoxifen is widely accepted by clinicians in the treatment of postmenopausal patients with hormone-sensitive breast cancer; its use in patients who have hormone-insensitive breast tumors and in premenopausal patients continues to be evaluated. Many physicians are currently prescribing the drug, but precisely who should receive it, the risks involved, and the actual benefits are still unclear.

Even more controversial is a new study in which healthy women who are at high risk of developing breast cancer, primarily because of a strong family history of the disease, are being given preventive tamoxifen. Whereas proponents suggest that the drug may reduce the incidence of breast cancer in such women by as much as 30 to 40 percent, critics claim that this figure is an overestimation. They do not wish to see healthy women exposed to the possibility of tamoxifen side effects, which in some circumstances can be life threatening, and recommend restricting use of the drug to women with known breast cancer.

Because there is no medical consensus on the use of tamoxifen in premenopausal patients, in those with hormone-insensitive tumors, or as a preventive agent in healthy women, the decision about this therapy is often left to the patient. In order to make sound judgments concerning her own treatment, the patient must be well informed about the potential risks and benefits of each type of therapy she is to receive. An individual without a medical background, or with little knowledge of medical jargon, is obviously dependent on her physician's ability to assess all treatment options accurately. The decision, however, should not be solely in the hands of her doctor. The patient must ask questions, learn about the different forms of treatment, and weigh the risks of each against its benefits.

Our purpose in this book is to educate women about the treatment and prevention of breast cancer in the hope that they can work with their doctors to decide the best possible treatment alternative. We begin by suggesting some of the questions a woman may want to ask her doctor if she has been diagnosed with breast cancer. We then briefly cover the types of surgeries she may be offered. We introduce the reader to drug therapy in breast cancer and emphasize systemic chemotherapy—how it works, how effective it is, and what its side effects are. In the remainder of the book we focus on the hormonal agent tamoxifen, perhaps the most disputatious therapy in the treatment of breast cancer. We cover its development, its use in breast cancer, its side effects, failures of tamoxifen treatment, and finally its controversial use in the prevention of breast cancer in healthy women.

We thank Vernon Emshoff and Greg Wurz for their help in preparing this manuscript. And we are grateful to the staff of Yale University Press for rapid and professional publication.

Tamoxifen and Breast Cancer

1

Common Questions
about Breast Cancer

A diagnosis of breast cancer is one of the greatest fears among women. Although such a diagnosis is cause for concern, the outcome is not necessarily fatal, particularly when the disease is caught in the early stages. In fact, early breast cancer is considered more than 90 percent curable by surgery alone. In the later stages, complete cures using surgery, radiation, and chemotherapy do occur; even when the cure is not complete, control of the disease may allow the patient to live for a long time.

Coping with breast cancer is not easy, but the fear and other intense emotions are more readily managed by learning about the disease. If you have been diagnosed with breast cancer, learn what you can from books and articles found in bookstores or the public library. Call the Cancer Information Service (1-800-4-CANCER) and the office of the American Cancer Society nearest to you. Demand to know all possible treatment alternatives. Recognize that the diagnosis was based on your physical examination and the pathology report. Therefore, the opinion of a second doctor—and in some cases a second pathologist—may be a good idea.

Remember that you are your best advocate; don't be afraid to ask for information. Questions not only help you to understand your disease, but they may ultimately increase your chances of getting the best possible treatment, which could lead to a cure. You must first research the disease and learn the types of questions to ask your doctor. The following suggestions are meant to guide you.

COULD THE LUMP I FOUND IN MY BREAST BE CANCER?

Ask the doctor what the lump could be and why he or she thinks so. Tell the doctor about any changes you have noted in your breasts, including pain or tenderness; differences in size or shape; dimpling, puckering, or retraction of the nipple; flaking skin on the nipple; or nipple discharge. If the doctor recommends a mammogram (a soft-tissue X-ray of the breast) and one is taken, find out what the results are. Ask how this mammogram compares to any previous ones that are available. Inquire if a biopsy should be made, and if not, why not.

Because the majority of lumps found in women's breasts turn out to be fibrocystic disease, do not panic if you find a lump. But do not put off seeing your doctor. The assumption that a lump in the breast is merely a noncancerous cyst is not only naive but may be extremely dangerous. Furthermore, if you have experienced long-term problems with cysts of the breasts (fibrocystic disease), do not accept a wait-and-watch approach if a new lump develops. Ask your doctor to biopsy the lump or, at the least, to arrange for another mammogram.

HOW CAN THE DOCTOR TELL IF A LUMP IS CANCER OR JUST A CYST?

It is not always easy for your doctor to distinguish between a cancerous lump and a cyst by means of a physical exam alone. But there are some distinctions. Cysts tend to fluctuate in size with the menstrual cycle, and are usually painful and sore. In contrast, a cancerous lump is apt to be more stable in size and less tender. Typically, cysts are easier to move, more spherical, and softer than breast tumors, which are anchored to surrounding tissues. Ask your doctor his or her impression of the lump. If a needle biopsy is performed, ask if the fluid or material recovered from the lump indicated a fluid-filled cyst. Often the size of a cyst will decrease once the fluid has been aspirated from it, so ask whether such a decrease in size has occurred.

A mammogram is another good tool in helping the doctor to decide if the lump is cystic or cancerous. Unfortunately, it is not foolproof and should be done in conjunction with a biopsy. The mammogram may show small calcifications (which show up as white densities) when cancer is present. In the case of cystic disease, larger calcifications may also be present. The shape and density of the lump tend to be the distinguishing factors: cysts generally have a very uniform density and may have a small surrounding ring of thick, fibrous tissue; tumors are much more irregular in shape and density.

WHAT KIND OF BIOPSIES ARE AVAILABLE?

Several types of biopsies can be performed, some of them on an outpatient basis (a needle biopsy, for example). Others are more complicated and require a longer recovery time. Ask your doctor which procedure will be performed, and determine whether a simpler procedure could provide the same results.

If your doctor is fairly certain that the lump is cancerous, he or she may suggest a biopsy at the time of the surgery to remove the tumor. This is called a one-step procedure, because the biopsy is performed right on the operating table. In most cases, however, the doctor will recommend a two-step procedure. The biopsy is performed first, and the surgery later if it is indicated. The pathologist thus has more time to examine the biopsied tissue carefully before a decision is made. You as patient also have more time to consider what kind of surgical procedure is acceptable.

IF THE BIOPSY SHOWS THAT I HAVE CANCER, WHAT IS THE NEXT STEP?

After a lump is diagnosed as cancerous, your doctor may order a variety of tests to make sure the cancer has not already spread to other parts of the body. Chest X-rays, bone scans, and liver function tests may be performed. Ask you doctor how big the tumor is, and whether any lymph nodes are involved. Has the cancer spread? The doctor may tell you the rating of the tumor according to specific definitions of tumor size and degree of spread to the lymph nodes (see table 1). In general, the lower the numbers, the easier the cancer will be to treat with surgery or chemotherapy (1).

Table 1. *Stages of Breast Cancer, as Determined by the International Union against Cancer*

Stage	TNM Classification*	Extent of Tumor
0	Tis, N0, M0	In situ (confined to lobules or ducts); has not spread below membrane of breast
I	T1, N0, M0	Small (greatest dimension < 2 cm); has not spread to lymph nodes of armpit or to other more distant areas of body
IIA	T0, N1, M0 or T1, N1, M0 or T2, N0, M0	2 cm or smaller and has spread to lymph nodes in armpit; or 2–5 cm but has not spread to lymph nodes of armpit
IIB	T2, N1, M0 or T3, N0, M0	2–5 cm and has spread to lymph nodes in armpit, but nodes are not attached to one another; or > 5 cm but has not spread to lymph nodes or other more distant areas of body

(continued)

Table 1 (*continued*)

Stage	TNM Classification*	Extent of Tumor
IIIA	T0, N2, M0 or T1, N2, M0 or T2, N2, M0 or T3, N1–2, M0	2–5 cm or smaller and has spread to several lymph nodes of armpit, causing adhesion to one another or to blood vessels; or > 5 cm and has spread to lymph nodes of armpit
IIIB	T4, N0–3, M0 or T0–4, N3, M0	Any size, but either is fixed to chest wall or muscle, or involves lymphatics of skin or skin itself and may or may not involve lymphatic nodes of armpit; or any size but has spread to lymph nodes above collarbone
IV	T0–4, N0–3, M1	Any size; lymph nodes may or may not be involved but cancer has spread to areas other than breast and lymph nodes

Source: Adapted from J. R. Harris, M. Morrow, and G. Bonadonna. Cancer of the breast. In *Cancer: Principles and Practice of Oncology,* V. T. DeVita, S. Hellman, and S. A. Rosenberg, eds. Philadelphia: J. B. Lippincott, 1993 (4th ed.), 1264–1332.

*T0 = no evidence of primary tumor; Tis = tumor in situ; T1 = tumor < 2 cm; T2 = tumor 2–5 cm; T3 = tumor > 5 cm; T4 = tumor any size, accompanied by involvement of chest wall; involvement of lymphatics within skin of breast; infiltration of skin by malignant cells; and skin ulceration.

N0 = no cancer present in lymph nodes; N1 = cancer involvement but nodes are movable; N2 = nodes attached to one another or to adjacent blood vessels; N3 = cancer spread to nodes above collarbone.

M0 = no metastasis; M1 = metastasis to distant site.

Ask the doctor what kind of breast cancer you have and how fast this sort of tumor grows. He may tell you that the cancer is in situ, meaning that it is confined to a very small area and has not yet formed a tumor mass. In situ breast cancers are readily treated, and because of their small size, are generally detected by mammography rather than biopsy. The doctor may also use the phrase "infiltrating breast cancer," which means that cancer cells which began growing in a milk duct or lobule have grown through the membrane of that duct or lobule and are now forming a tumor in the surrounding tissues.

You should also ask if estrogen or progesterone receptors were present in the tumor, and if hormonal therapy is an option. The presence of such receptors means that there are proteins inside the cancer cells that bind the estrogen and progesterone. Once these hormones bind, the cell is stimulated to grow. These hormone-sensitive cells are easier to treat than cells that lack hormone receptors (known as hormone-insensitive cells). If the hormone receptors are present, the doctor is likely to prescribe a hormonal therapy, such as tamoxifen, which blocks the estrogen receptor and prevents the stimulation of cell growth. Ultimately the growth of hormone-sensitive breast cancer cells is thereby retarded.

It is important that a number of other tests be performed on the tumor specimen. The pathologist looks at the primary genetic material, or DNA (deoxyribonucleic acid), of the breast cancer cells to determine if it is abnormal in appearance or quantity and to see how many cells are in the process of dividing or active growth (2). This determination of how aggressive (or fast growing) the tumor is helps to predict how you as a patient will fare in the long term (see table 2). It may also aid the doctor in choosing the proper type of chemotherapy and indicate how well you will respond to such treatment.

WHAT KINDS OF SURGERIES ARE AVAILABLE?

At one time most women with breast cancer were given few choices about the extent of surgery that could be performed to remove a breast cancer. Today there are many choices, and they are not

Table 2. *Pathology Findings and Meaning for Patient's Prognosis*

Finding	Resulting Prognosis
Estrogen receptors	Good
Progesterone receptors	Good
Diploid DNA	Good
Haploid DNA	Bad
High S-phase (percent)	Bad

Source: Adapted from D. E. Merke and W. L. McGuire. Ploidy proliferative activity and prognosis: DNA flow cytometry of solid tumors. *Cancer* 65: 1194–1206 (1990).

always easy. Although the doctor may make recommendations, the final decision is often left to the patient. She therefore needs to be well informed on what types of surgery are available and the advantages and disadvantages of each. She should ask her doctor for a definition of each type of surgery, the amount of tissue that will be removed, the potential for reconstructive breast surgery, the additional therapy that may be necessary, and the risk of cancer recurrence following the surgery. In actuality, the surgical cure rate is strongly dependent on the stage of breast cancer diagnosed in the patient. At stage I, the cure rate is 90 to 100 percent; at stage II, 60 to 90 percent; at stage III, 20 to 30 percent; and at stage IV, it is 0.

There are two types of surgery, a lumpectomy and a partial mastectomy, that do not remove large portions of the breast. In a lumpectomy, only the cancerous lump is excised—although the doctor may also remove a number of axillary lymph nodes (in the armpit on the same side as the breast lump) to check for the spread of cancer. In a partial mastectomy, the cancerous lump and some of the normal tissues surrounding it are removed. Again, several lymph nodes in the armpit are removed and checked for cancer. Both surgeries tend to be good options for large-breasted women with small tumors; they avoid total breast amputation, reduce the pain and discomfort associated with the more extensive operations, cause less destruction of muscle tissue, and induce less swelling subsequent to surgery. For smaller-breasted women these procedures are not always a satisfactory option, in that removal of a portion of the breast may significantly change its size or shape. This type of surgery is also inappropriate for women with multiple cancerous lumps or women whose tumors involve the underlying muscle.

If your doctor recommends either of these operations, ask how many of them he or she has performed. Will the doctor be removing any lymph nodes to check for the spread of cancer; if not, how can he or she be sure that the cancer has not spread to the lymph nodes? How disfiguring will the surgery be? Is the risk that the cancer will spread any greater with the chosen procedure?

Typically, both of these surgeries are followed by radiation therapy, a treatment that helps reduce the likelihood of cancer recurrence and is considered necessary postsurgical follow-up. The initial radiation treatment is given over a 30-minute period daily for four to six weeks. A subsequent treatment, a few weeks later, consists of daily dosages for approximately a week. If you will undergo radiation therapy, be aware of the added time and expense, and discuss these matters with your doctor when considering your options.

The doctor may suggest a mastectomy instead of these less invasive procedures. In this surgery the entire cancerous breast is removed. The doctor's selection of this alternative will be based on several factors: the size of the tumor, its location, the type of tumor, the size of your breasts, and whether the cancer has spread to the lymph nodes or elsewhere. If your doctor recommends a mastectomy, several further options must be considered. They differ primarily in the amount of other normal tissue (muscle, lymph nodes, fat) that is removed in addition to the breast itself. The most common variants are simple mastectomy, modified radical mastectomy, and radical mastectomy.

A simple mastectomy removes the entire breast but leaves the underlying muscle tissue intact. Typically, a number of lymph nodes are removed to check for the spread of cancer.

A modified radical mastectomy is a common procedure that

removes the entire breast including the tissue lining over the muscles of the chest, and sometimes the muscle itself. The lymph nodes of the armpit are taken out, which may lead to some swelling after surgery. A modified radical mastectomy is frequently used to treat women with early-stage breast cancer, particularly those whose breasts are medium to small in size.

A radical mastectomy is by far the most disfiguring surgery and is performed much less frequently than the other two operations. This surgery removes the breast, the muscles of the chest that support the breast, the fatty tissue of the chest and armpit, and all the lymph nodes of the armpit. The patient is left with reduced muscle strength in the arm, significant pain and swelling, and major disfigurement of the chest.

Should your doctor suggest any of these procedures, ask about the degree of disfigurement that may result, and about the potential for reconstructive surgery later on. In general, the more tissue that remains, the easier the reconstructive surgery will be. Therefore, reconstructive surgery following a radical mastectomy can be rather difficult. If your doctor has recommended a radical mastectomy, ask if it is absolutely necessary. Consider getting a second opinion, preferably from a surgical oncologist associated with a large medical center. Most physicians today believe they can achieve equivalent results by performing a much less extensive modified radical mastectomy.

WHAT KIND OF SURGERY SHOULD I HAVE?

The type of surgical procedure performed is generally based on the stage of breast cancer noted at diagnosis (table 1). For women who have stage 0 breast cancer, which is confined to the lobules or the ducts, many doctors prefer the safest approach and recommend a total mastectomy, particularly for small-breasted women. Some physicians will bypass removal of the lymph nodes of the armpit; others prefer to remove them to make certain the cancer does not spread. For women with larger breasts, the doctor may suggest a lumpectomy or a partial mastectomy, followed by radiation therapy. You should be aware that there is a small but statistically significant difference in the rate of cancer recurrence. The cure rate following a simple mastectomy is essentially 100 percent, whereas the rate of cancer recurrence has been shown to increase about 1 percent each year after a lumpectomy with radiation.

For women with stage I or II breast cancer, the rate of cure following a simple mastectomy is not 100 percent; it has been shown to be approximately equivalent to the rate subsequent to the less extensive surgical procedures. Many doctors therefore suggest a lumpectomy or partial mastectomy in these instances. Still, a doctor may recommend a simple mastectomy to some patients—those, for instance, with multiple tumors, a large tumor, tumors that have spread to the lymph nodes, or tumors that involve the center of the breast.

Table 3. *Risk Factors for Developing Breast Cancer*

Major Risk Factors
    Previous breast cancer
    Age over 50
    Strong family history of breast cancer
        (1) If two first relatives (mother, daughter, or sister) have had breast cancer, risk is 5 to 6 times average
        (2) If one aunt, grandmother, or cousin has had breast cancer, risk is 1.5 times average

Minor Risk Factors
    Onset of menstruation at age 12 or younger
    Onset of menopause after age 55
    No children, or first child after age 30
    Breast cysts or precancerous breast disease

Unproven but Potential Risk Factors
    High fat diet (> 20 percent of calories consumed)
    Obesity
    Alcohol (moderate to heavy consumption)
    Radiation exposure
    Pesticides and other environmental pollutants
    Estrogen replacement therapy in postmenopausal women with strong family history of breast cancer

---

In stages III and IV breast cancer the tumor is generally much larger and may require chemotherapy to shrink it prior to surgery. After the tumor has responded to treatment, surgery is performed to remove as much as possible of the remaining tumor in the breast. The operation may be a modified radical mastectomy or, in some cases where the tumor has spread to other parts of the body, a lumpectomy may be performed.

WHO IS MOST LIKELY TO DEVELOP BREAST CANCER?

Many factors are known to be associated with the development of breast cancer (see table 3). The most important risk factors appear to be (1) a previous diagnosis of breast cancer in one breast, (2) age over 50, and (3) a mother, daughter, or sister who has had breast cancer, particularly if she was premenopausal. Other risk factors include onset of menstruation at age 12 or younger, onset of menopause after age 55, no children or birth of children late in life (after age 30), and a history of breast cysts or precancerous breast disease.

IS HEREDITY A RISK FACTOR?

Heredity does appear to be a strong influence in the development of breast cancer. The risk of developing the disease increases five-fold or sixfold if at least two first relatives (mother, daughter, or sister) has had the disease. This risk is greater if the cancer was diagnosed as premenopausal or was detected in both breasts. If a second-degree relative (aunt, grandmother, cousin) had breast cancer, the risk is increased by only 1.5 times the average. Heredity, however, may involve more than the genetic predisposition to develop the disease.

Other risk factors, including dietary and environmental influences, may arbitrarily be "handed down" in families or cultures (3). Although there is no direct association in humans between breast cancer and a fatty diet, studies suggest that a high-fat, high-calorie diet may increase the incidence of tumor development in animals

(4). Dietary factors also have been significantly associated with increased incidence of breast cancer in Japanese women who have emigrated to the United States. Japanese women living in Japan traditionally have had very little breast cancer; their diet is low in fat and high in fiber. Unfortunately, after emigration to the United States the incidence of breast cancer in these women has increased threefold until it has approached the rate for U.S. women. Other western cultural changes may be involved, including later pregnancies and increased exposure to environmental hazards (5).

WHAT ARE THE HORMONAL RISK FACTORS?

Hormonal influences are extremely important. Long-term exposure to estrogens has been shown to increase the incidence of breast cancer in animals and women. In some species of animals such as the dog, the risk of developing breast cancer increases with each menstrual (estrous) cycle. In women, we have seen that those who begin menstruation at an early age or who experience menopause late also have an increased risk of breast cancer. Women whose ovaries have been removed or who enter menopause at an early age are less likely to develop breast cancer (1). Although most physicians do not believe that estrogens are a direct cause of breast cancer, they may act to stimulate the growth of cancer cells that are already present.

WHAT ARE THE ENVIRONMENTAL RISK FACTORS?

Environmental hazards are perhaps the least-understood risk factors associated with breast cancer. We do know that exposure to repeated low or modest levels of radiation increases the risk of developing breast cancer. Women who have received upper-body radiation or multiple X-ray procedures may be at increased risk. But repeated single diagnostic procedures and repeated mammograms involve only low doses of radiation and at this time are considered insignificant as risk factors.

Other environmental causes are speculative. Exposure to high-voltage electrical power lines or appliances (electromagnetic radiation) is currently being evaluated as a possible underlying cause of many forms of cancer, such as childhood leukemia and brain cancer. In most of these cases, the children have been found to live or play near a power substation or high-voltage overhead lines. Further studies are required before any direct association can be made between electromagnetic radiation and a variety of cancers, including breast cancer.

It has become evident that pockets of breast cancer exist in certain geographic areas, such as Long Island, New York. Environmental factors may be involved, because most of the women who are afflicted do not have other risk factors. Whether affluent women have different dietary habits, tend to bear children later in life, incur increased exposure to electromagnetic radiation from multiple household appliances, or experience unknown environmental toxins (such as pollutants in drinking water or pesticides) remains uncertain. To date, the studies evaluating the high-risk pockets have failed to demonstrate an environmental cause for the higher incidence of breast cancer documented in these areas.

Recent media reports suggest that exposure to at least one environmental toxin (the pesticide DDT) may be linked to a fourfold increase in the incidence of breast cancer. This subject requires further scientific research. Because many environmental toxins accumulate in fish and animal fat, avoidance of fish from areas known to be polluted and a diet low in animal fat may help to reduce the risk of exposure to toxins. Although the use of DDT has been banned by the government for years, its long-term effects are only now being recognized. The cancer-causing potential of pesticides and other chemical products in use today may be hidden for years to come. Utilization of environmentally friendly products—and prudent use of all chemicals—may help to alleviate at least some of the risk for future generations.

Although many of the elements mentioned above have been associated with breast cancer, it is important to remember that only one-third of the women who develop breast cancer have known risk factors (6). In addition, although family history of breast cancer is high on the list of risk factors, approximately 75 percent of the women who develop breast cancer have no such history.

2

Drug Therapy

Following surgery and perhaps radiation therapy, most patients feel a sense of relief that their cancer is gone and they can resume their normal lives. Yet often there is one last hurdle: treatment with chemotherapy or hormone therapy to prevent recurrence of the cancer. There is a measure of contradiction in the administration of harmful drugs at a time when the patient is just beginning to feel healthy. The short-term toxic effects (such as loss of hair) seem particularly devastating at this stage, but the lifesaving value of these agents over the long term is vastly more important.

DO I NEED SYSTEMIC CHEMOTHERAPY?

For many women with breast cancer, surgery is followed by chemotherapy administered into the bloodstream over several cycles. The need to receive chemotherapy may be confusing to the patient: Why should further treatment be given if the tumor has been removed? In general, surgery is very successful in getting rid of the initial cancerous growth. Tumor cells, however, can spread

to other parts of the body such as the lymph nodes, internal or-
gans, or bone—where they may not be detected until much later.
Chemotherapy effectively reduces the risk that new tumors will
arise from these hidden, potentially cancerous cells; studies have
shown that it may diminish the likelihood of recurrent breast cancer in women by 20 to 37 percent (7). Unfortunately, there is a
definite time frame in which the chemotherapy must be given in
order to achieve optimal results, and this "window of opportunity"
comes soon after surgery. Chemotherapy at this time has the ad-
vantage that tumor cells are still limited in number and have not
developed into a full-blown tumor. Although chemotherapy is not
very appealing to a patient so soon after the trauma of surgery,
timely administration is crucial.

WHAT ARE THE DIFFERENCES BETWEEN
CYTOTOXIC SYSTEMIC CHEMOTHERAPY
AND HORMONAL THERAPY?

The drugs used in cytotoxic chemotherapy differ from hormonal
agents in many ways, and their effects on cancer cells are substantially different. In general, cytotoxic drugs work by killing the
cancer cells, whereas hormone therapy works by stabilizing cancer
cell growth. The complete destruction of cancer cells, resulting in
cell death, gives rise to the term "cytotoxic" drug. Conversely,
therapy with hormones such as tamoxifen is said to be "cytostatic"
in nature, which means that it inhibits cells from dividing further
but does not kill them. Because the drugs used in chemotherapy
are directly toxic to cells, they are given over a short period of time.
In contrast, hormonal agents need to be present at all times in
sufficient quantity to inhibit or block the growth of cancer cells.
Thus, tamoxifen and similar substances must be taken on a daily
basis rather than for just a few doses or cycles.

Chemotherapy also tends to be toxic to normal cells. Even
though some of the toxicities can be alleviated by adjusting the
dosage, the range of doses within which the drug (or drugs) must
be given in order to achieve an antitumor effect without also producing serious damage is extremely narrow. If not enough drug is

given, or if the cancer cells are no longer sensitive to chemotherapy, patients may experience many of the side effects of chemotherapy but fail to respond to the treatment. On the other
hand, if too much of a cytotoxic drug is given, the patient may have
a satisfactory tumor response but risk more severe toxicities, some
of which could be life threatening.

WHICH CYTOTOXIC DRUGS
ARE GIVEN SYSTEMICALLY?

A variety of cytotoxic agents have been found to be effective in the
systemic treatment of breast cancer (1). The most commonly used
drugs are listed in table 4. Typically, these agents are not used
alone but in combination with one another or with other sub-

Table 4. *Major Chemotherapy Drugs Used in Breast Cancer*

Drug (generic name)	Other Name(s)	Method of Application*
Cisplatin	Platinum, Platinol	IV
Cyclophosphamide	Cytoxan, Endoxan	IV, PO
Doxorubicin	Adriamycin	IV
5-fluorouracil	5-FU, Adrucil	IV
Melphalan	Alkeran, phenyl-alanine mustard	PO
Methotrexate	Amethopterin, Mexate, Folex	IV, PO, SC, IA, IT
Mitomycin	Mutamycin	IV
Triethylene thio-phosphoramide	Thiotepa	IV, IM, SC, IT
Vinblastine	Velban	IV
Vincristine	Oncovin	IV

*IA = intraarterial (injected in artery)
 IM = intramuscular (injected in muscle)
 IT = intrathecal (injected in space surrounding spinal cord)
 IV = intravenous (injected in vein)
 PO = oral (given by mouth)
 SC = subcutaneous (injected under skin)

stances. Not all cancer cells are in the same phase of cell division at a given time; thus, some cells may be sensitive to a specific drug while other cells are resistant. To attain maximum benefit from chemotherapy it is vital to use an assortment of drugs that can act on different phases of cancer cell growth. Three categories of systemic drugs typically are used to treat breast cancer: natural products (such as anthracyclines and vinca alkaloids), alkylating agents, and antimetabolites. The categories are differentiated based on the way in which the drugs act to kill cancer cells. Drugs may be selected from each category and used separately or in combination.

Anthracyclines   Doxorubicin (trade name Adriamycin), commonly used in the treatment of breast cancer, is a member of a group of antibiotics that are produced by bacteria called streptomyces. Although its exact mechanism of action is poorly understood, doxorubicin appears primarily to interfere with the copying of the primary genetic material DNA before the cell divides.

Vinca Alkaloids   The vinca alkaloids include vinblastine and vincristine. These agents are derived from the periwinkle, or vinca plant, and act on cancer cells by interfering with some of the machinery involved in cell division (specifically, the mitotic spindle). The cell can then no longer replicate or copy its genetic material, and it dies in the process of division. Vinca alkaloids are also known as phase-specific agents, because they work on a particular phase of the cell growth cycle. They are most effective in cancer cells that are rapidly dividing, such as those found in newly developing tumors. Unfortunately, these drugs affect normal cells too, so that prolonged use can result in some degree of toxicity to the nervous system, or neurotoxicity.

Alkylating Agents   Alkylating agents are synthetic drugs that are believed to function by interfering with a number of cellular processes: copying of the genetic material (replication), converting the cellular information into readable form (transcription), and processing the information into protein (translation). When such interference takes place, cells can no longer reproduce their genetic material—which is a requirement for continued growth. Cyclophosphamide is an example of an alkylating agent. It is commonly used in breast cancer treatment, usually in combination with other drugs such as methotrexate and 5-fluorouracil. This "CMF regimen" was developed by the National Cancer Institute and reportedly has a response rate higher than 50 percent in breast cancer patients. Cyclophosphamide is a phase-nonspecific drug, meaning that its effectiveness does not depend on the rapid division of the cells. It can therefore be used in tumors with slow growth rates (advanced tumors, for example).

Antimetabolites   Methotrexate and 5-fluorouracil are both classified as antimetabolites. In general, the chemical structure of antimetabolites is similar to that of the cellular metabolites normally found within a cell. These agents can fool the cell by incorporating themselves into the cellular pathways that are involved in synthesizing materials necessary for cell growth. Both agents interfere with the making of DNA, RNA (ribonucleic acid), and proteins, an action that prevents further growth and replication of the cancer cell.

WHAT ARE THE SIDE EFFECTS OF THESE DRUGS?

Among the primary concerns of patients requiring treatment are the various side effects associated with systemic cytotoxic chemotherapy. Yet the majority of these reactions are temporary. Many side effects, such as nausea and vomiting, last only hours or days. In addition, although each drug has multiple toxicities, the patient will rarely experience all the adverse effects of any one agent. Furthermore, the development of new ways to treat nausea and vomiting, and to aid in the recovery of bone marrow, has significantly reduced the incidence and severity of the side effects of many chemotherapy drugs.

The principal cause of side effects is that the drugs involved affect not only cancer cells but normal cells—especially those characterized by rapid growth. These include cells of the hair follicles, mouth, stomach, and bone marrow. The bone marrow is composed of very fast growing cells that are busily dividing in order to make new red cells, white cells, and platelets. These blood cells eventually work their way into the bloodstream. The red cells carry oxygen to all the tissues of the body; the white cells are part of the immune system, which helps in wound healing and allows the body to fight off infection; the platelets assist in forming blood clots in damaged tissues. Chemotherapy on cells of the bone marrow can generate serious side effects, including a decrease in red cells causing anemia, a decrease in white blood cells potentially enhancing the risk of infection, and a reduction in the number of platelets thus causing bleeding or clotting problems.

The side effects of each drug have been well documented (see table 5), but unfortunately they are not usually predictable. Some

Table 5. *Possible Side Effects of the Major Chemotherapy Drugs*

Drug	Common Side Effects	Less Frequent Side Effects
Cisplatin	Nausea and vomiting, bone marrow suppression	Bone marrow depression, kidney and neurologic problems, hearing loss
Cyclophosphamide	Nausea and vomiting	Bladder problems, bloody urine, lung problems, skin discoloration, hair loss, secondary cancers
Doxorubicin	Nausea and vomiting, burning at injection site, hair loss, bone marrow depression, red color of urine	Liver, heart, kidney problems; skin discoloration; skin reactions; fever; mouth sores

(continued)

Table 5   (*continued*)

Drug	Common Side Effects	Less Frequent Side Effects
5-fluorouracil	Nausea and vomiting, bone marrow suppression	Diarrhea, mouth sores, hair loss, skin discoloration, nail problems
Melphalan	Nausea, bone marrow suppression	Lung problems, hair loss, secondary cancers, menstrual irregularities, mouth sores
Methotrexate	Bone marrow suppression, nausea, diarrhea	Gastrointestinal, liver, kidney problems; mouth sores; headache; fever; hair loss
Mitomycin	Nausea and vomiting, burning at injection site	Bone marrow depression, diarrhea, fever, lung and kidney problems, hair loss, fatigue, mouth sores, eye problems
Thiotepa	Nausea and vomiting, bone marrow suppression	Fever, allergic reactions, dizziness
Vinblastine	Burning at injection site, bone marrow suppression	Nausea and vomiting, headache, hair loss, diarrhea, constipation, mouth sores, loss of reflexes, mental depression

(*continued*)

Table 5   (*continued*)

Drug	Common Side Effects	Less Frequent Side Effects
Vincristine	Burning at injection site, hair loss	Bone marrow suppression, nerve damage (sharp pain or tingling in extremities, loss of reflexes), constipation, mental depression

patients experience only mild symptoms; other women receiving the same drugs and dosages experience severe toxicities. Physical and psychological variables exert an influence as well.

WHEN SHOULD THESE DRUGS BE GIVEN?

In the case of systemic chemotherapy, the ideal time to initiate treatment is within a month of surgery. Regrettably, a single dosage is not sufficient to assure the total elimination of cancer cells. Your doctor will usually recommend several cycles of treatment, primarily in the hope that all cancer cells will be killed in serial treatments. The number of treatments, and whether or not radiation is administered concurrently, depends on the extent of the tumor. Breast cancer that has spread to other areas, or is large in size, may require more cycles of therapy than a small tumor that has not spread to surrounding tissues.

WHICH DRUGS ARE GIVEN IN COMBINATION CHEMOTHERAPY?

One of the most commonly used drug combinations in breast cancer is the CMF regimen that uses cyclophosphamide, methotrexate, and 5-fluorouracil. Many oncologists consider this the standard treatment for breast cancer that has metastasized to the lymph nodes. For patients requiring less aggressive therapy, the cyclophosphamide may be eliminated. For patients needing slightly more aggressive therapy, adriamycin may be given instead of methotrexate. Because adriamycin is more potent and has more side effects than methotrexate, it is reserved for more aggressive therapies. Regimens using adriamycin may also include cyclophosphamide and 5-fluorouracil; they are then known as CAF or FAC.

Vincristine and prednisone may be added to CMF if still more aggressive therapy is required. For patients with advanced disease, a combination of cyclophosphamide, adriamycin, and vincristine (CAV) or of vinblastine, adriamycin, thiotepa, and the hormonal agent halotestin (VATH) may be administered.

Alternating treatment programs, such as CMF combined with VATH, or high-dose regimens may also be given. As yet, few studies have evaluated the order of drugs given in alternating regimens; however, it appears likely that the sequence may make a difference. In one study by Bonadonna and colleagues (8, 9) an improvement in disease-free survival (the length of time the patient is free of disease from diagnosis until tumor recurrence) and in overall survival (the length of time the patient survives following diagnosis) was noted in patients receiving adriamycin followed by cyclophosphamide, methotrexate, and 5-fluorouracil.

WHY NOT USE JUST ONE DRUG?

For many years it was acceptable practice to treat breast cancer with only one type of drug. Single agents including 5-fluorouracil, cyclophosphamide, and melphalan were shown to improve disease-free survival rates over surgery alone. Still, none of the clinical trials using single agents resulted in uniform improvement in the overall survival rates of breast cancer patients. In contrast, clinical trials using combination chemotherapy have demonstrated consistent improvement in both disease-free and overall survival rates for premenopausal patients, and modest improvement for postmenopausal patients (see table 6).

Table 6. *Reduction in Breast Cancer Recurrence and Mortality Following Combination Chemotherapy or Tamoxifen*

Treatment*	Age (years)	Menopausal Status†	Reduction in Recurrence (% ± S.E.)	Increase in Survival (% ± S.E.)
TAM	< 50	Pre	12 ± 4	6 ± 5
CC	< 50	Pre	36 ± 5	25 ± 6
TAM	< 50	Post	12 ± 15	—
CC	< 50	Post	37 ± 19	—
TAM	50–59	Pre	33 ± 7	23 ± 9
CC	50–59	Pre	25 ± 9	23 ± 9
TAM	50–59	Post	28 ± 3	19 ± 4
CC	50–59	Post	29 ± 5	13 ± 7
TAM	60–69	Post	29 ± 3	17 ± 4
CC	60–69	Post	20 ± 5	10 ± 6
TAM	70+	Post	28 ± 5	21 ± 6
CC	70+	Post	—	—

Source: Adapted from Early Breast Cancer Trialists' Collaborative Group. Systemic treatment of early breast cancer by hormonal, cytotoxic, or immune therapy. *Lancet* 339: 1–15, 71–85 (1992).

*CC = combination therapy
 TAM = tamoxifen
†Pre = premenopausal
 Post = postmenopausal

It is now known that the use of several drugs together is more effective than one drug alone in eliminating the cancer. Because each type of drug works on cancer cells in a different way, when the drugs are used together there is a greater chance that if some cells have escaped the lethal effects of one drug, they will succumb to the toxicity of the other agents. Some drug combinations therefore have a synergistic effect. In other words, the combination of drugs works better at killing the cancer cells than the additive effect of the individual drugs.

Combination chemotherapy may also limit the side effects generated by one drug alone. The side effects of some drugs depend on the total dosage. Combination therapy permits lower doses of each individual drug, thus reducing the potential for dose-dependent side effects.

HOW MUCH CHEMOTHERAPY SHOULD BE GIVEN?

The amount of chemotherapy is dependent on a number of factors, including the health of the patient, the stage of the disease at diagnosis, the aggressiveness of the tumor, and the patient's tolerance of any prior chemotherapy. In general, smaller doses are given to patients with a history of liver, kidney, or heart disease, and to patients diagnosed in the very early stages of breast cancer. Lower dosage is also given to elderly patients or to those patients who have had significant side effects from previously administered chemotherapy. If the cancer has only been diagnosed in its late stages, or if the tumor is considered aggressive, then larger doses are administered. High-dose regimens, long-term therapy, or alternation of drug combinations may be utilized in the case of extremely aggressive tumors. The interval between cycles may also be altered so that the chemotherapy is administered more frequently than at the customary intervals of three to four weeks.

HOW LONG SHOULD CHEMOTHERAPY BE GIVEN?

In early breast cancer clinical trials, most treatment protocols continued chemotherapy for one to two years. Studies using fewer courses of chemotherapy showed similar results, suggesting that long-term administration may not provide further benefits. Current investigations suggest that chemotherapy should be given for at least three months in order to achieve maximum benefit (7). In addition, analysis of repeated treatments using the same drug combination suggests that benefits cease at six cycles. Therefore the optimal number of cycles appears to be six (7, 10). Nevertheless, the intervals between cycles can be changed, or the length of treatment extended, depending on the specific characteristics of the patient.

WHAT ABOUT VERY HIGH DOSE CHEMOTHERAPY PLUS BONE MARROW TRANSPLANTATION?

Bone marrow transplantation is a relatively new approach to the treatment of breast cancer and is still considered experimental by many physicians. The procedure was originally developed for the treatment of patients with leukemia (cancer of the blood system), lymphoma (cancer of the lymphatic system), and other blood disorders. Very high doses of chemotherapy not only killed the cancer cells but also resulted in the death of normal cells in the bone marrow. Patients could then be "rescued" by bone marrow transplantation (that is, by implanting new bone marrow cells from a healthy person, usually a relative). While this strategy is now acceptable for the treatment of many diseases, it is still considered a high risk procedure.

Bone marrow transplantation relies on extremely high doses of drugs that may have significant and sometimes long-term side effects. Liver and kidney damage as well as lasting neurological problems may result. Short-term problems are also possible, for the bone marrow is destroyed in the procedure and the newly transplanted marrow may take time to rejuvenate. The use of new agents called colony stimulating factors, which activate the new bone marrow, have helped to reduce the time during which a patient is susceptible to infections and bleeding complications.

Other long-term side effects, such as rejection of the transplanted bone marrow cells, have been eliminated by means of autologous bone marrow transplantation. The patient's own bone marrow is collected or "harvested" from her pelvis or hipbone before she receives any chemotherapy. The harvested marrow is stored until it is needed. The patient receives very high doses of chemotherapy in the hope of killing all the cancer cells. In the process, the patient's normal bone marrow cells are also destroyed. Her own bone marrow cells can then be returned to her via injection into the vein. Surprisingly, these cells work their way back into the bone, where they begin to reseed the depleted bone marrow.

Since the patient's immune system recognizes the transplanted bone marrow as "self," rejection is not a problem.

Owing to the use of autologous bone marrow and the development of agents that help to bolster the immune system following transplantation, the dangers of bone marrow transplantation have been significantly reduced. Still, the procedure is not without risk. In general, it is reserved for patients where breast cancer has spread to distant sites, particularly when more than ten lymph nodes are involved.

3

Tamoxifen
and How It Works

The antiestrogenic agent tamoxifen, touted by some as a miracle drug, is currently the most widely prescribed hormonal agent used for the treatment of breast cancer. Although it cannot take the place of systemic chemotherapy, tamoxifen does provide a less toxic alternative in patients unable to tolerate the side effects of systemic chemotherapy. Effective alone and in combination with systemic chemotherapy, tamoxifen is primarily used in postmenopausal patients with hormone-dependent (estrogen-receptor-positive) breast cancers. But in recent years its role has expanded to include all ages and hormone receptor statuses. Its exact role in the treatment of breast cancer continues to be controversial. As a result, patients are often uncertain whether they should be receiving the drug. The following chapters discuss the information currently available on tamoxifen and its role in the treatment and prevention of breast cancer.

Tamoxifen, commercially available since the mid-1970s, is a synthetic nonsteroidal compound (fig. 1). It has hormone-like effects, however, and can act to block estrogen receptors. Tamoxifen was

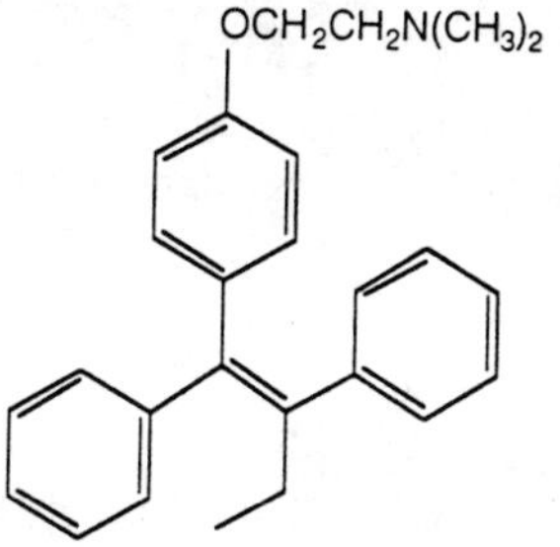

OCH$_2$CH$_2$N(CH$_3$)$_2$

Fig. 1. Chemical structure of tamoxifen.

first made in 1966 by scientists at the Imperial Chemical Industries in Great Britain (11). They were attempting to synthesize agents that could be used for birth control. Although tamoxifen was successful for this purpose in some animals, in mammals it was found to be less effective than many other agents (12, 13). Because it was also observed to block the effects of estrogens (or to have anti-estrogenic effects), it was then studied as a potential breast cancer therapeutic agent.

WHAT WAS THE RATIONALE BEHIND THE USE OF TAMOXIFEN IN THE TREATMENT OF BREAST CANCER?

The treatment of breast cancer in the early 1960s was primarily limited to chemotherapy. While such agents are very effective, they do also have a significant number of side effects—many of which are related to the fact that they are active against fast-growing cells. Thus, fast-growing cells other than cancer cells may be incidental targets for these toxic drugs, particularly cells of the hair follicles, bone marrow, and gastrointestinal tract. This fact triggered interest in alternative and less toxic therapies for breast cancer.

By the 1960s it had become evident that at least some forms of breast cancer were dependent on hormones for growth, specifically on the steroid hormone estrogen. Evidence for this association originated almost a century ago, with the observation that in

some women surgical ovariectomy (removal of the ovaries) caused shrinkage or remission of breast cancers (11). Much later evidence showed that some types of breast cancer were dependent on estrogen for growth. With removal of the ovaries—the primary source of estrogen in women—estrogen levels were reduced, causing inhibition of breast cancer cell growth. Agents that blocked the effects of estrogen proved to be equally effective in the treatment of estrogen-receptor-positive breast cancer.

IS TAMOXIFEN A GOOD ALTERNATIVE TO CHEMOTHERAPY?

Evaluation of the use of antiestrogenic agents, including tamoxifen, to treat breast cancer began in the late 1960s. Because most antiestrogens temporarily arrest or slow the growth of estrogen-dependent breast cancer cells and have no apparent effect on breast cancer cells that are not estrogen dependent, there was only modest interest in using these agents, particularly for the treatment of advanced breast cancer in premenospausal patients. Because of the low incidence of side effects compared to chemotherapy, though, tamoxifen has become a satisfactory alternative to cytotoxic chemotherapy, particularly in individuals who cannot tolerate the rather harsh side effects of chemotherapy. From experience we now know that tamoxifen may be used as an alternative to chemotherapy in many patients and may even be used in conjunction with it.

HOW DOES TAMOXIFEN WORK?

Many questions relating to how tamoxifen inhibits the growth of breast cancer cells remain unanswered. For years tamoxifen was assumed to act simply by blocking the effects of estrogen on breast cancer cells (14). It is recognized that some types of breast cancer cells contain proteins called estrogen receptors. When estrogen, which normally is synthesized in the ovaries and carried by the bloodstream, comes in contact with cells carrying these estrogen receptors, the estrogen binds with the receptors in a way that trig-

gers the growth of these cells. If estrogen can be removed from the system (for example, when the ovaries are removed), then these receptor-positive cancer cells are no longer stimulated to grow. Furthermore, if drugs can be given that interact with the estrogen receptors without stimulating cell growth, then the cell is blocked from the growth-triggering effect of estrogen even in the presence of estrogen. Although a variety of other mechanisms are currently under investigation (15), it appears that the mechanism by which tamoxifen inhibits breast cancer growth is at least in part related to its binding and blocking of the estrogen receptor.

IS TAMOXIFEN MORE EFFECTIVE IF ESTROGEN RECEPTORS ARE PRESENT IN THE TUMOR?

Over the years numerous scientific investigators have been able to isolate estrogen receptors from breast cancer cells and demonstrate their binding to estrogen, as well as the blockage of such binding by tamoxifen. Estrogen receptors consist of amino acids that are linked together to form a protein. A receptor-positive cell contains many hundreds or thousands of these receptors, which are located in the nucleus, near where the genetic information is stored. They are also present in the cytoplasm, where much of the cell's work is performed. Estrogen receptors have been found in cells other than breast cancer tissues. They occur in many normal cells including the bone, the liver, the endometrium (lining of the uterus), and normal breast tissue.

The ability to isolate estrogen receptors led to the further study of this protein and to the development of a method to measure the content of estrogen receptors in breast cancer tissues. This technique helped physicians to determine which patients are most likely to benefit from the use of tamoxifen. Although the earliest diagnostic tests were relatively crude and often led to false results, the estrogen receptor tests utilized today offer much more accurate results. If the presence of estrogen receptors is detected in biopsy tissue taken from a cancerous breast, then tamoxifen has a substantial chance of being effective.

CAN TAMOXIFEN WORK EVEN IF NO
ESTROGEN RECEPTORS ARE PRESENT?

The absence of estrogen receptors in breast cancer cells does not always imply that a patient will not respond to tamoxifen. There is evidence that tamoxifen also inhibits 8 to 15 percent of hormone-independent or estrogen-receptor-negative breast cancer cells (16). Some physicians report responses in patients who supposedly are estrogen receptor negative; however, the doctors believe that these patients probably do have estrogen receptors that for some reason are not being detected, either because of their low number or perhaps because they are functionally different in some way from normal estrogen receptors. Alternatively, the clinical responses noted in these patients have led some to believe that tamoxifen may also work by some mechanism other than blockage of the estrogen receptor.

In fact, several groups of researchers have demonstrated that there may be more than one kind of estrogen receptor (17, 18). Receptors that differ from the normal type are called variant estrogen receptors. Some appear to result when a normal gene for a receptor is erroneously copied, first into a messenger-RNA variant and then into a variant receptor protein with altered or defective function. Other variant estrogen receptors have been identified, suggesting that they may occur in many forms. If their presence in certain patients is not recognizable by current techniques, this fact would explain why some estrogen-receptor-negative patients nevertheless benefit from tamoxifen.

CAN TAMOXIFEN WORK ON PARTS
OF THE CELL OTHER THAN
THE ESTROGEN RECEPTOR?

Recent research suggests that tamoxifen can interact with cells to alter the amount of the activity of substances called growth factors (19). These are proteins produced and secreted by certain types of cells, which act to stimulate or inhibit the growth of breast cancer cells. It appears that tamoxifen can induce the production of at

least one kind of growth factor from stromal cells (20), which are normal cells that surround cancerous cells in the breast tissue. The secreted protein is called transforming growth factor-beta (TGF-β).

Other studies suggest that tamoxifen is broken down in the liver to several different compounds known as tamoxifen metabolites. At least one of these metabolites, 4-hydroxytamoxifen, is more effective than tamoxifen and is thought to be responsible for the majority of tamoxifen's activity in inhibiting breast cancer cell growth. Although, like tamoxifen, this metabolite binds to estrogen receptors, it has also been found to bind very tightly to other cellular proteins. These proteins are called antiestrogen binding sites, or AEBSs (21), and their function remains poorly understood. Further research may show that they too are involved in tamoxifen's ability to inhibit the growth of breast cancer cells.

4

Tamoxifen
in Breast Cancer

In the late 1960s it was common practice to offer irradiation of the ovaries at the time of initial treatment of breast cancer to all premenopausal women, including women within three years of probable menopause. We have seen that irradiation of the ovaries essentially destroys the ability of the ovaries to make estrogen, thereby reducing levels of that hormone in the blood. For patients with recurrent breast cancer or metastatic cancer (beyond the breast tissue and local lymphatic system), hormone therapy was often instituted: premenopausal patients were prescribed androgens with or without cytotoxic drugs; postmenopausal patients were prescribed estrogens. It was unclear what form of hormone therapy should be offered to patients presumably within five years of menopause. The reaction of this group to hormone therapy was very poor. Alternative therapies were therefore needed to improve both overall response rates and the treatment of premenopausal women.

WHEN WAS TAMOXIFEN FIRST USED?

Because most of the original information about tamoxifen was derived from animal studies, many questions had to be addressed concerning the subset of patients who would benefit from the drug, the length of treatment, the amount of drug needed, and the requisite frequency of administration. Most of the early clinical trials were conservative in design and were initiated primarily in elderly postmenopausal patients who had not tolerated chemotherapy well (22).

In the early 1970s the results of the first trials of tamoxifen for the treatment of breast cancer were published. Response rates were reported to be on the order of 20 to 22 percent, which was comparable to results from other forms of hormone therapy in use at the time (23–25). The incidence of major side effects from tamoxifen was much lower, however, and the drug was effective in patients who did not respond to other forms of hormone therapy —suggesting that there was no cross resistance between hormonal agents. Interestingly, the best responses were noted in women in their fifties who were within three years of expected menopause (perimenopausal). This was the population that had previously been insensitive to hormone therapy, so tamoxifen gave them a new alternative.

WHEN DID TAMOXIFEN BECOME
STANDARD TREATMENT?

In 1977 tamoxifen was approved by the Food and Drug Administration (FDA) for use in the treatment of breast cancer, initially only in postmenopausal women with metastatic breast cancer. Of this population approximately one-third responded to tamoxifen treatment. When used in addition to chemotherapy for patients with metastatic disease, a higher response rate, a longer time to treatment failure, and improved survival were reported (1, 11). In postmenopausal patients tamoxifen appeared to be effective at virtually all stages of disease, with its major contribution in patients who had exhausted most other forms of hormonal therapy.

HOW DOES TAMOXIFEN COMPARE
TO OTHER HORMONAL AGENTS?

Several randomized clinical trials have been performed on tamoxifen in postmenopausal patients in order to compare it to other hormonal agents. In one trial tamoxifen was compared to diethylstilbestrol (DES), which during the 1970s was considered the standard initial treatment for postmenopausal patients with breast cancer. Results from these trials were similar to the initial pilot studies and suggested that tamoxifen had approximately the same response rate (31 percent) as DES (33 percent). Both the frequency and the incidence of side effects were much lower in the tamoxifen group (23–25). In subsequent clinical trials comparing tamoxifen to several alternative surgical procedures to reduce estrogen levels, tamoxifen produced approximately the same response rates but without the dangers associated with the surgical forms of therapy (26, 27).

More recently, tamoxifen was compared with another hormonal agent, aminoglutethimide, as treatment for postmenopausal breast cancer patients. Aminoglutethimide acts on the adrenal gland to reduce the amount of estrogen-like substances synthesized and secreted. Again, tamoxifen produced a comparable response rate without many of the side effects produced by the comparison substance (28).

IN WHAT PATIENT POPULATION IS
TAMOXIFEN MOST EFFECTIVE?

Further evaluation in postmenopausal patients led to the conclusion that tamoxifen is most effective in patients with tumors that are estrogen dependent. This judgment was confirmed following the development of assays that measure estrogen receptors in breast cancer specimens, making it possible to establish which patients would be most likely to benefit from tamoxifen therapy. Patients with estrogen-receptor-positive tumors are considered to have a better chance of responding to tamoxifen than those with estrogen-receptor-negative tumors.

On the average, tamoxifen produces response rates of 50 percent or higher in postmenopausal patients with estrogen-receptor-positive tumors, as compared to rates of about 10 percent in those with estrogen-receptor-negative tumors (29). Additional factors are associated with an improved likelihood of responding to tamoxifen: previous response to other forms of hormonal therapy; long duration (years) between initial diagnosis and recurrence of breast cancer; and metastatic breast cancer confined to bone, lung, or soft tissue (1, 11).

WHO SHOULD RECEIVE SYSTEMIC CHEMOTHERAPY OR HORMONAL THERAPY?

Premenopausal versus Postmenopausal Patients   We have seen that the decision about whether to treat with systemic chemotherapy or hormonal therapy is dictated by a number of factors, which include the size of the tumor at diagnosis, menopausal status, and the degree to which the cancer has spread to other areas such as the lymphatic channels and axillary nodes. From numerous studies performed since the mid-1970s, we know that systemic chemotherapy is very effective in reducing the risk of cancer recurrence, particularly in premenopausal patients. Hormonal therapy has been substantially less effective in this population (see table 6).

Originally, premenopausal women were excluded from studies evaluating the efficacy of tamoxifen in breast cancer. It was believed that the high circulating levels of estrogen in their blood would interfere with tamoxifen's ability to block the estrogen receptor. Several clinical trials evaluating tamoxifen's use in premenopausal patients have shown response rates of up to 30 percent, however, which is approximately the response rate observed following removal of the ovaries in such patients (15, 30, 31). In estrogen-receptor-positive premenopausal patients, the response rate is higher; approximately 40 percent of the patients responded (26), a rate consistent with the results achieved by ovariectomy in this group.

Thus recent trials indicate that tamoxifen may be a satisfactory

alternative to surgical ovariectomy in premenopausal patients, particularly in the setting of advanced or metastatic disease. Adjuvant tamoxifen may also significantly reduce the risk of breast cancer recurrence in premenopausal patients, but to date significant improvement in overall survival has been observed only in patients older than 50 years.

In postmenopausal patients, the efficacy of systemic chemotherapy in prevention of breast cancer recurrence has been controversial. Most physicians feel that patients of this age should receive more effective forms of hormonal therapy, particularly if their tumor tissue contains either estrogen or progesterone receptors. Increasing evidence indicates, however, that some postmenopausal patients benefit from the use of certain systemic chemotherapy combinations. In this group of patients, both systemic chemotherapy and hormonal agents may be used in combination.

In summary, systemic chemotherapy is most often used in premenopausal patients, whereas hormonal therapy is more commonly used in postmenopausal patients. Combination therapy (hormonal plus systemic chemotherapy) can be used in both populations, however.

Patients with Node-Positive and Node-Negative Breast Cancer   Chemotherapy was first shown to be effective in patients with breast cancer that had spread to the axillary lymph nodes. This form of treatment appears to be most effective in patients who have one to three positive nodes, but is also beneficial to those with four or more involved nodes. In "node-negative" patients (in whom the cancer has not yet spread to the lymph nodes), most cures are by surgery or other forms of local therapy alone. But approximately 20 to 30 percent of node-negative patients may develop a breast cancer recurrence and eventually die of metastatic disease. It is difficult to determine who in this subset of patients is most at risk for recurrence and therefore most likely to benefit from chemotherapy. In general, patients who have invasive tumors greater than one centimeter in diameter are given systemic chemotherapy. Factors that may increase the risk of recurrence include a very large tumor at initial diagnosis, estrogen-receptor-negative status,

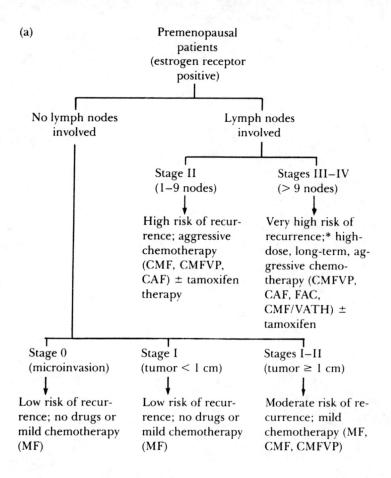

(a)

Premenopausal patients (estrogen receptor positive)

No lymph nodes involved

Lymph nodes involved

Stage II (1–9 nodes)

→ High risk of recurrence; aggressive chemotherapy (CMF, CMFVP, CAF) ± tamoxifen therapy

Stages III–IV (> 9 nodes)

→ Very high risk of recurrence;* high-dose, long-term, aggressive chemotherapy (CMFVP, CAF, FAC, CMF/VATH) ± tamoxifen

Stage 0 (microinvasion)

→ Low risk of recurrence; no drugs or mild chemotherapy (MF)

Stage I (tumor < 1 cm)

→ Low risk of recurrence; no drugs or mild chemotherapy (MF)

Stages I–II (tumor ≥ 1 cm)

→ Moderate risk of recurrence; mild chemotherapy (MF, CMF, CMFVP)

Fig. 2. Current trends in the treatment of premenopausal patients with breast cancer: (a) estrogen-receptor-positive patients and (b) estrogen-receptor-negative patients.

Notes: See Chapter 2 for definitions of the various chemotherapies and Chapter 1 for definitions of the stages.

BMT = bone marrow transplantation
CAF = cyclophosphamide, adriamycin, and 5-fluorouracil
CMF = cyclophosphamide, methotrexate, and 5-fluorouracil
CMF/VATH = cyclophosphamide, methotrexate, and 5-fluorouracil alternating with vinblastine, adriamycin, thiotepa, and halotestin

(b)

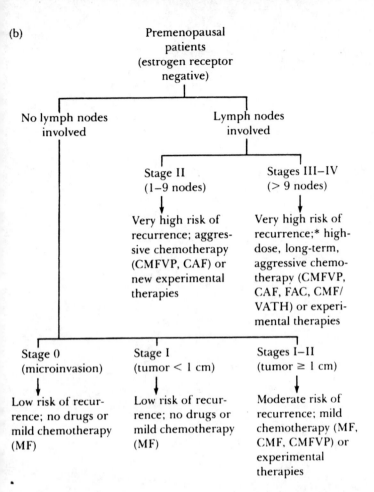

Fig. 2 (*continued*)

CMFVP = cyclophosphamide, methotrexate, 5-fluorouracil, vincristine, and prednisone (or prednisolone)

FAC = 5-fluorouracil, adriamycin, and cyclophosphamide

FAC/VATH = 5-fluorouracil, adriamycin, and cyclophosphamide alternating with vinblastine, adriamycin, thiotepa, and halotestin

MF = methotrexate and 5-fluorouracil

*In stage IV, cancer has already spread beyond the breast and lymph nodes.

(a)

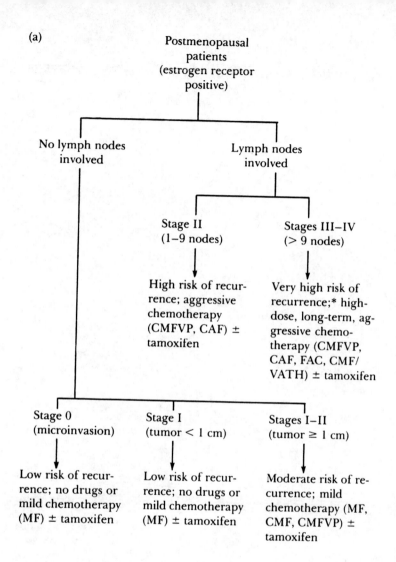

Fig. 3. Current trends in the treatment of postmenopausal patients with breast cancer: (a) estrogen-receptor-positive patients and (b) estrogen-receptor-negative patients.
Notes: See figure 2.

(b)

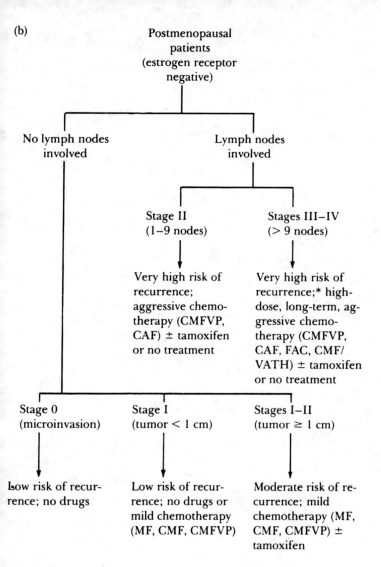

and a tumor that is identified by the pathologist as aggressive (poorly differentiated) or rapidly proliferating. Typically, tumors with a large number of cells that are actively dividing (a high percentage of cells in S-phase) are considered more aggressive than tumors with a low fraction of cells in S-phase (7; see also table 2).

Tamoxifen's role in the treatment of breast cancers that are in situ (preinvasive) or that have minimal (microscopic) invasion beyond the ducts or lobes is still being debated. Most physicians feel that the risk of tumor recurrence after surgery in this group of patients is relatively low and that it is not worth the risk of potential side effects from chemotherapy. Current clinical studies using tamoxifen in patients with estrogen-receptor-positive tumors that are node negative suggest that tamoxifen is effective in reducing recurrence regardless of patient age.

Patients Who Are Estrogen Receptor Positive   In general, an estrogen-receptor-positive patient will be offered tamoxifen, particularly if she is postmenopausal. If a patient has cancer that has spread to the lymph nodes, chemotherapy may also be given. Some oncologists prescribe tamoxifen for patients who are estrogen receptor negative. While it cannot be determined with assurance which patients should receive which form of therapy, the current trends for premenopausal and postmenopausal women are shown in figures 2 and 3.

WHY NOT GIVE CHEMOTHERAPY AND
TAMOXIFEN TO EVERY PATIENT?

It must be kept in mind that for each patient the benefits from either chemotherapy or tamoxifen therapy must be weighed against the risks and costs. The benefit in many cases may translate into a delay in tumor recurrence, not a cure. The side effects of chemotherapy can be life threatening, and these risks are easily weighed against chemotherapy's life-prolonging effect. The side effects of tamoxifen are less common and not as life threatening, so that it is more difficult to weigh risks against benefits. Obviously, though, the life-prolonging effects are achieved with much less

toxicity than those produced by chemotherapy. In patients with a tumor smaller than one centimeter, the absolute benefit from tamoxifen therapy is small—approximately 2 percent fewer tumor recurrences. Compared to the incidence of tamoxifen-induced side effects such as life-threatening thromboembolic disease (1.5 percent risk) or endometrial cancer (1.1 percent risk), the benefit from tamoxifen therapy may not be worth the risk (32–38). Furthermore, tamoxifen must be taken daily for two to five years at a cost of up to a thousand dollars per year (in the United States). The long-term side effects more than ten years after a course of tamoxifen of more than two years are also unknown.

SHOULD CHEMOTHERAPY BE GIVEN AT THE SAME TIME AS TAMOXIFEN?

Since most tumors are a mixture of estrogen-receptor-positive and estrogen-receptor-negative cells, and tamoxifen specifically inhibits cells with estrogen receptors, combination therapy using both cytotoxic drugs and tamoxifen has been suggested to prevent the recurrence of the estrogen-receptor-negative cells (see Chapter 2). Clinical trials examining the simultaneous use of chemotherapy and tamoxifen suggest that the drugs probably should not be given at the same time. Although higher response rates were achieved in some studies when the drugs were given together, most analyses have shown that the overall survival of patients is not prolonged by simultaneous administration.

WHAT ABOUT SEQUENTIAL CHEMOTHERAPY AND TAMOXIFEN?

The administration of cytotoxic chemotherapy followed by tamoxifen has been examined in several programs. Sequential administration appears to avoid the problems noted when the drugs are administered simultaneously. Patients treated sequentially seem to have fewer residual side effects from chemotherapy during tamoxifen treatment, which may ultimately improve their quality of life. Sequential use has also been demonstrated to be very effective in

the treatment of metastatic breast cancer. In advanced disease the sequential addition of tamoxifen to chemotherapy results in some patients having a higher response rate, a longer time until treatment failure, and improved overall survival.

5

Side Effects of
Tamoxifen

When reviewing the side effects of any drug, we need to remember that some may occur very frequently, whereas others are extremely rare. In addition, a given individual may experience no side effects at all from the therapy or she may experience the full range. It is important to keep in mind that many side effects can be alleviated, or at least made tolerable, if brought to the attention of the physician.

WHAT IS THE INCIDENCE
OF SIDE EFFECTS?

The incidence of tamoxifen side effects is quite small compared to most other chemotherapeutic agents used in the treatment of breast cancer. It is a comparison of apples and oranges, however. Most patients who receive chemotherapy have active or advanced disease, whereas tamoxifen is usually given to patients who are judged free of disease. Therefore, any adverse effects of tamoxifen would be considered to significantly affect the quality of a patient's life. Most of the side effects are related to tamoxifen's antiestrogenic activity, although the drug is known to have some estrogenic effects as well. For the most part, tamoxifen has been particularly well tolerated in clinical trials, with only a handful of patients (3 to 4 percent) having to withdraw because of acute adverse effects (14). Overall, the incidence of hormone-related side effects is much lower in postmenopausal patients. In premenopausal patients, tamoxifen may produce symptoms similar to menopause, with menstrual irregularities occurring in as many as 20 to 35 percent of patients (15).

WHAT ARE THE MOST
FREQUENT SIDE EFFECTS?

The most common side effect of tamoxifen is hot flashes (see table 7). Directly related to the antiestrogenic and partial estrogenic effects of tamoxifen, these have occurred in as many as 10 to 20

Table 7. *Side Effects of Tamoxifen Therapy*

Side Effect	Incidence
Hot flashes	10–20 percent
Nausea and vomiting	10 percent
Constipation or diarrhea; loss of appetite	Rare
Vaginal bleeding/discharge/dryness/itching	Occasional
Tumor flare reaction*	Rare
Fluid retention/weight gain	2–16 percent
Disturbances of the central nervous system†	Occasional
Thrombocytopenia	2 percent
Ocular toxicity	Rare
Secondary endometrial tumors	0.17–1.7 percent
Secondary liver problems or tumors	Unknown

*Includes increase in pain, swelling or erythema, and increased serum calcium levels.

†Includes dizziness, depression, nervousness, fatigue, lethargy, and irritability.

percent of patients studied (15). Menstrual irregularities, vaginal bleeding, and vaginal dryness or itching have all been reported. Mild nausea with or without vomiting occurs in about 10 percent of patients (1, 11). Other gastrointestinal problems including loss of appetite, constipation, and diarrhea have also been reported (39). Edema (water retention) and weight gain take place in 2 to 16 percent of patients (31, 40).

DOES TAMOXIFEN CAUSE ANY OF THE PSYCHOLOGICAL SYMPTOMS ASSOCIATED WITH MENOPAUSE?

Tamoxifen does produce a number of other symptoms similar to those noted during menopause. It has been associated with depression or irritability in some patients, whose signs may go largely ignored by physicians. Dizziness or light-headedness, nervousness, headache, fatigue, and lethargy have all been noted (41–43). Additional studies are needed to define the incidence of psychological side effects.

WHAT IS MEANT BY A FLARE REACTION?

Tamoxifen has been associated with a reaction known as tumor flare. Soon after initiation of tamoxifen treatment there may be an apparent increase or flare in tumor size and symptoms including bone or tumor pain and swelling and redness of the area around the tumor (44, 45). New lesions may develop. This condition is most often seen in patients who have breast cancer involving the bones, and it is also associated with a rise in blood calcium concentration (hypercalcemia; 14, 46). It is therefore important to monitor the first few weeks of tamoxifen therapy very closely in patients with breast cancer. In most instances, the high calcium levels are transient or can be treated with appropriate drugs; the tamoxifen need not be discontinued. In fact, for many patients the tumor flare reaction is often followed by a positive tumor response to tamoxifen.

WHAT EFFECT DOES TAMOXIFEN
HAVE ON THE BONE MARROW?

Tamoxifen has a mild suppressive effect on the bone marrow of approximately 2 percent of patients (43). A slight decrease in the number of platelets and both red blood cells (those cells involved in blood clotting and oxygen transport) and white blood cells (those involved with fighting infection) has been reported. While side effects of tamoxifen are rare, doctors should occasionally monitor patients' blood counts, particularly when dealing with long-term administration of the drug.

ARE THERE ANY LIFE-THREATENING
SIDE EFFECTS?

Most of the typical side effects of tamoxifen are not considered life threatening. Still, there have been rare reports of thromboembolic disease involving either phlebitis or venous thrombosis in patients taking tamoxifen. Phlebitis is an inflammation of the wall of the blood vessel that makes the vessel weak and prone to clotting and obstruction. Venous thrombosis is the formation of a blood clot in the vein. Blood clots that develop in the large veins of the arms, legs, or trunk may be very serious if not treated immediately. In one multicenter clinical study a significant increase in thromboembolic disease was observed in patients receiving tamoxifen versus patients receiving a placebo (47; table 8). Although thromboembolic disease need not be life threatening in itself, it can lead to pulmonary embolism. Pulmonary emboli are blood clots that travel to the lung, obstructing its blood flow and producing a potentially catastrophic emergency.

Although thromboembolic disease is considered a rare side effect of tamoxifen therapy, its incidence is approximately ten times that noted with estrogen therapy. In fact, the incidence of thrombophlebitis with oral contraceptive therapy (1 in 2,000 women) is considered a significant risk to healthy women. Because the incidence of tamoxifen-induced thrombophlebitis is on the order of 1.5 in 100 women, this side effect has perhaps been downplayed.

Table 8. *Increased Incidence of Thromboembolic Disorders in Patients Taking Tamoxifen*

| Disorder | Severity | Number of Patients Affected in Group Taking | |
		Tamoxifen	Placebo
Superficial phlebitis	Mild	3	0
Vein thrombosis	Moderate	4	0
Deep-vein thrombosis	Severe	6	2
Pulmonary embolism	Life threatening	6	1
Death		2	0
Total incidence (total number of patients)		21(1,422)	3(1,440)
Percent incidence		1.5	0.2

Source: Results reported by the National Surgical Adjuvant Breast and Bowel Project (NSABP) B-14.

The symptoms of thromboembolitic disease include leg or arm swelling, pain, and warmth; or abrupt shortness of breath, chest pain, and cough, with spitting up of blood. Any patient experiencing these symptoms should consult her doctor immediately. In most cases, she can easily be treated by administering blood-thinning drugs such as heparin or warfarin that help to dissolve the existing clots and prevent further coagulation.

CAN TAMOXIFEN CAUSE LIVER CANCER?

Preclinical animal studies have shown that tamoxifen may in fact act as a weak promoter of liver cancer. In rats fed low doses of tamoxifen, liver tumors occurred in approximately 11.5 percent of the animals, and at higher doses as many as 71.2 percent developed liver cancer (48). To date there have been only anecdotal reports of a possible association between liver cancer and the use of tamoxifen in humans. Remember, however, that we know very little about the long-term side effects of this drug when it is given

for more than five years. Furthermore, because breast cancer in its advanced stages frequently metastasizes to the liver, some liver cancers potentially caused by tamoxifen could be incorrectly attributed to the spread of breast cancer. The result would be an underestimation of the actual incidence of liver cancers attributed to tamoxifen (6). Liver biopsies are potentially useful in determining whether a cancer in the liver is chemically induced by tamoxifen or is a result of breast cancer cells that have metastasized.

Although no direct link to liver cancer has been made, accounts of liver complications from tamoxifen are on the rise. Reports from a Committee on the Safety of Medicines in the United Kingdom suggest that at least four deaths have occurred in five patients who developed liver failure from tamoxifen. At least one other death occurred among five patients with tamoxifen-induced hepatitis (49).

WHAT EFFECTS DOES TAMOXIFEN HAVE ON THE UTERUS?

Over the years there has been growing evidence that tamoxifen induces tumor growth in the lining of the uterus (or endometrium). In a recent study many of the women who developed irregular vaginal bleeding due to tamoxifen therapy were found also to have small noncancerous growths or polyps of the uterine lining (34). A number of them went on to develop tumors of the endometrium.

Although many physicians consider the incidence of tamoxifen-induced uterine tumors to be small, there is still a significant risk (33, 50, 51). In one clinical study evaluating 46 nonhysterectomized postmenopausal women receiving tamoxifen for 6 to 36 months, 13 patients developed noncancerous growths or polyps, 8 had thickening of the uterine lining, and 2 developed cancer of the endometrium.

The incidence of uterine tumors appears to increase with higher doses of tamoxifen (34). With the usual dose of 10 mg twice daily, an incidence of 0.17 percent was reported, while patients receiving

20 mg of tamoxifen twice daily had an incidence nearly ten times higher (1.2 percent).

Although surgical hysterectomy can be performed once a tumor develops in the uterus, new evidence suggests that the types of tumors that develop while a woman is taking tamoxifen are extremely aggressive. Women who develop uterine cancers induced by tamoxifen therapy may be more likely to die from uterine cancer than those who spontaneously develop this form of cancer (52).

CAN TAMOXIFEN CAUSE EYE PROBLEMS?

Tamoxifen has been associated with the development of eye problems in some patients. Typically, most individuals who developed eye problems received high daily doses of tamoxifen—120 mg twice a day (53). In recent studies, however, eye problems including both corneal and retinal changes have been reported in 6.3 percent of patients receiving much lower tamoxifen doses—20 mg twice daily (54). These changes may or may not be associated with decreased visual acuity and are not always corrected when tamoxifen is discontinued. Because this side effect is more commonly found in patients receiving high doses of tamoxifen or prolonged courses of therapy, periodic eye examinations should be performed.

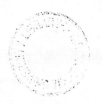

6

Tumor Recurrence and Tamoxifen Resistance

Fortunately for many women, once an initial tumor has been detected and surgically removed, there is little chance of tumor recurrence. With the use of radiation, systemic chemotherapy, or tamoxifen the risk of recurrence may be further reduced. A number of women, however, will have tumors that recur either locally (in the treated breast or breast wall) or at a distance (in the form of metastatic disease).

At one time the fear of tumor recurrence led many physicians to advocate radical mastectomies or modified radical mastectomies to patients initially diagnosed with breast cancer, in the hope of eliminating the tumor totally and preventing tumor recurrence. We now know that lumpectomies or partial mastectomies often are equally effective in completely removing the primary tumor.

If another breast cancer develops after a lumpectomy or partial mastectomy, it may be a recurrence of the original tumor or it may be a new and unrelated cancer. If such a tumor develops on the chest wall outside the normal breast tissue or adjacent to the mastectomy site, it is likely that the original cancer has recurred.

Unfortunately, there is then a high risk that the cancer will spread to other parts of the body.

WHERE DOES BREAST CANCER SPREAD?

When breast cancer does recur outside the breast, it usually does so in rather specific areas. One of the most common locations is in the bone. Although the bones of the ribs, spine, pelvis, and upper arms and legs are most commonly involved, breast cancer can metastasize to virtually any skeletal area. This process may be heralded by local bone pain or ultimately bone fracture, but painless bone metastases are common as well.

The spread of breast cancer to the lymph nodes is also quite prevalent. The lymph nodes adjacent to the breast and under the arm, called "axillary nodes," are the most frequently affected areas. Breast cancer may also spread to the liver and lungs or throughout the skin and into the brain.

IS TUMOR RECURRENCE OUTSIDE
THE BREAST TREATABLE?

Breast cancer that occurs outside the breast is treatable, but is generally much harder to cure than local recurrence. Physicians try to design treatments that will provide the patient with the best possible chance of curing the disease while avoiding additional risk in terms of life-threatening side effects. Therapy given to control tumor symptoms when there is little hope of cure is called palliative.

HOW IS RECURRENT BREAST
CANCER TREATED?

For breast cancer that has recurred within the initially treated breast, an aggressive type of surgery is usually performed. If the earlier surgery was a lumpectomy or partial mastectomy, a complete mastectomy may now be required. Once the tumor and surrounding tissues have been removed, the tumor will be evaluated for the presence of estrogen and progesterone receptors. The decision to use chemotherapy, radiation, or hormone therapy will be based on the size and location of the tumor, nodal involvement, the presence or absence of receptors, and the prior use of chemotherapy drugs. For tumors considered to place the patient at high risk of recurrence, or when conservative surgery is performed, radiation is used subsequently to decrease the risk of another recurrence. As discussed earlier, for patients who have estrogen or progesterone receptors in their primary breast tumors, tamoxifen or another hormonal agent may be prescribed to control or prevent further tumor recurrence. Chemotherapy is also considered, depending on the kind of chemotherapy the patient received initially and how well she responded at that time.

If the breast cancer has spread to a single site outside the breast, treatment depends largely on where the tumor is located. If the recurrence is in an area that is surgically operable and the tumor impairs the patient's normal functioning, then the tumor may be surgically removed. For tumors of the bone or other tumors that are not readily operable, radiation may be used to reduce tumor size and alleviate symptoms.

Chemotherapy is typically given to patients with rapidly progressing or receptor-negative breast cancer that has spread beyond the breast. At one time it was believed that patients with disseminated breast cancer had little chance of long-term response to chemotherapy. Drugs were given primarily to moderate the symptoms of the disease. Today we know that by using different chemotherapeutic combinations an improved quality of life can be achieved in at least 60 percent of these patients.

As discussed in Chapter 2, most beginning drug therapies will include either methotrexate or adriamycin. Once a patient no longer benefits from the first protocol, she may be given a different course of drugs. Typically, a patient responds to the initial course for 6 to 12 months. When she stops reacting to any of the conventional drug combinations, the patient may elect to take a new and untested drug or combination of drugs that seems promising. Some of these agents have had encouraging results in patients with advanced breast cancer.

A patient with estrogen-receptor-positive breast cancer that has metastasized may be offered tamoxifen therapy before chemotherapy. Response to tamoxifen in patients with bone or soft-tissue metastasis is very good, and remission can last more than 12 months. Unfortunately, while response to tamoxifen may be as high as 75 percent in some groups, virtually all patients will eventually develop tamoxifen resistance and no longer respond. Once tamoxifen therapy fails to be effective, other hormonal agents such as aminoglutethimide, halotestin, megestrol, and leuprolide are available. As with tamoxifen, patients may initially respond satisfactorily, but eventually they develop resistance to all endocrine agents as well.

WHAT DOES IT MEAN IF THE DOCTOR SAYS MY BREAST CANCER IS NOW DRUG RESISTANT?

Drug resistance is a term used to describe a condition in which cells are able to survive despite drug therapy. There are at least two forms of resistance. In the first variety, called innate resistance, tumor cells are resistant even before any drugs have been given. This kind of resistance is usually not typical of breast cancer but is apt to be found in cancers of the kidney or lung. The second type is called acquired resistance, a condition whereby the cells actually "acquire" resistance following exposure to drugs. The cancer cells are very sensitive to the drugs at first, then become progressively less so. This sort of resistance is most often found in breast cancer. Although patients may at first respond very well to agents such as methotrexate or adriamycin, eventually the drugs stop working because of drug resistance.

HOW DOES THE DOCTOR KNOW THAT I HAVE DRUG-RESISTANT BREAST CANCER?

During your regular examinations, your doctor keeps track of how well your breast cancer is responding to the drugs that you have been given. Results from your physical exam, mammography,

X-rays, scans, biopsies, and a variety of blood tests are evaluated to see if the disease is improving, staying the same, or getting worse. When the results show that the tumor is getting larger or has spread to new areas even though you are taking chemotherapy, your doctor may assume that the tumor is no longer responding to the drugs currently being administered. At this point the doctor may suggest to you that your breast tumor is drug resistant. In this situation he or she may either increase the dose of drug to see if the tumor responds to the higher amount or change the type of drugs being administered.

WHAT CAUSES DRUG RESISTANCE?

Cancer cells develop resistance to specific types of drugs in many ways. Perhaps one of the first steps is exposure of the cells to concentrations of drug that are not high enough to kill them. A patient may have been given a dose of chemotherapy that is too low, or a standard dose may have been administered to a patient who has faster metabolism or excretes drugs more rapidly than the average person. Thus, the cells are exposed to low concentrations of drug without being killed. The resulting cancer cells are now "educated" about how to deal with the drug, so that even if the next dose is higher, the cells have a better chance of fending off its toxic effects. That is why chemotherapy drugs must be given in doses that are high enough to kill the cancer cells but below the level that causes severe side effects.

Once cancer cells have been exposed to a specific drug in concentrations that have not killed it, the cells may develop a number of techniques to handle the drug and keep themselves from being killed. Perhaps the most common mechanism that breast cancer cells adopt is the ability to pump the drug outside the cell (55, 56). This action occurs even in normal cells, where it functions to protect the cells from toxins during everyday life (dietary or environmental toxins, for instance).

Cancer cells have other methods of becoming drug resistant. In the case of methotrexate they actually go through elaborate changes in their biochemistry after exposure to the drug. The cancer cells have the ability to increase the amount of protein that is the target for methotrexate—an enzyme called dihydrofolate reductase. With augmented production of the enzyme, the cells have found a way to protect themselves from the lethal effects of the chemotherapy agent.

IS TAMOXIFEN RESISTANCE THE SAME PROBLEM?

Typically, most patients with breast tumors that are estrogen and progesterone receptor positive will respond to tamoxifen. When they develop resistance to tamoxifen after six months to a year of therapy, the tumor will begin to recur. Fortunately, for many patients who no longer respond to tamoxifen therapy another effective hormonal agent can be found. These alternative agents usually work for a period of time not exceeding a year, after which the patient again develops resistance. Tamoxifen tends to be given as a "first-line" therapy because it has significantly fewer side effects than other hormonal agents, so the development of resistance to this drug is a significant clinical problem.

At one time it was thought that a patient who no longer responded to tamoxifen probably was not taking the drug as directed (thus not enough drug was getting into the breast tumor cells) or perhaps was eating a diet high in "phytoestrogens." These are estrogenic compounds found in many plant products that were believed to stimulate the growth of breast cancer cells just as estrogen does (57, 58). The phytoestrogens are known to be capable of diminishing the effects of the antiestrogen tamoxifen. Weight gain over a prolonged period was also suspected to contribute to the loss of tamoxifen effectiveness (59). Because tamoxifen is a drug that is taken up by the fat cells and often retained in fatty tissue, an increase in weight without an increase in tamoxifen dose was believed to decrease the amount of drug available to the breast tumor. Even though all these explanations are plausible, their overall contribution to tamoxifen resistance is now considered minimal. Tamoxifen resistance apparently is associated with resistant mechanisms at the level of the breast cancer cell itself.

WHAT MAKES A CELL RESISTANT
TO TAMOXIFEN?

Many cellular changes have been associated with the development of tamoxifen resistance, but we still do not fully understand the basis of this clinical problem. After prolonged tamoxifen exposure a selection process may favor cells that have no estrogen receptors or cells that produce abnormal or aberrant receptors that fail to recognize tamoxifen (17, 18). Because tamoxifen is known to have estrogenic effects, scientific studies have shown that estrogenic metabolites of tamoxifen may contribute to the development of cellular resistance to tamoxifen (15, 59, 60). As in other types of drug resistance, there may be some form of cellular pump that removes tamoxifen from the cell.

Other research has focused on the involvement of proteins known as growth factors. Because tamoxifen is understood to increase the release from certain cells of the growth-inhibitory factor known as TGF-β, tamoxifen resistance may also occur when these cells can no longer produce the TGF-β required to continue restraining growth of the breast cancer cells (20, 61).

Much of this new information is speculative, yet it does suggest that several different mechanisms may contribute to the development of tamoxifen resistance. All require further investigation.

IF MY BREAST CANCER RECURS,
SHOULD I STOP TAKING TAMOXIFEN?

If a breast tumor continues to grow or a new tumor develops either in the breast or elsewhere while you are taking tamoxifen, it is probably best to discontinue the drug. One of the most important questions your doctor may ask before you stop is whether you have taken the drug as prescribed. If you have missed only a few doses, the doctor can reasonably assume that the tumor is no longer responding to the drug and has become resistant to tamoxifen therapy. If, however, you have taken the tamoxifen only sporadically, missing days or even weeks at a time, your doctor may elect to continue tamoxifen for a while to see if daily dosage will slow the growth of the tumor. Noncompliance in the tamoxifen regimen or prolonged absence of drug administration has contributed to tumor recurrence in some patients. It is therefore extremely important that you take tamoxifen exactly as prescribed and that you answer your physician's questions as accurately as possible.

IS THERE ANY HARM IN CONTINUING TO TAKE TAMOXIFEN EVEN IF MY DOCTOR RECOMMENDS STOPPING?

Perhaps one of the most alarming findings in the study of tamoxifen resistance is the evidence in humans and animals that after continued exposure to tamoxifen, tumors may actually become dependent on the drug for growth. The process is poorly understood and is being studied primarily in laboratory animals. Estrogen-receptor-positive tumors are grown in mice; when the animals are given tamoxifen, the tumors initially shrink. After about six months of continuous tamoxifen administration, however, the tumors begin to grow again. This time frame is approximately the same as is observed for the development of tamoxifen resistance in humans. Of further interest is the preliminary observation that if tamoxifen is given to mice for up to five years, then stopped, and estrogen is administered instead, the tamoxifen-resistant tumors disappear. It appears that the tumors not only avoid the inhibitory action of tamoxifen but somehow become dependent on it for continued growth (62, 63).

This evidence and other data on prolonged exposure of cells to tamoxifen suggest that breast cancer cells under conditions of long-term tamoxifen exposure can in fact learn to depend on the drug for growth and even be stimulated by it. Because these findings have been noted in laboratory studies on cultured cells and in animals, extrapolation to human patients is controversial. Nevertheless, several clinical studies have shown that in some women whose breast cancers began growing in the presence of tamoxifen, discontinuing the tamoxifen can itself produce a tumor stabilization or tumor regression (64, 65).

CAN TAMOXIFEN RESISTANCE BE PREVENTED?

Although a number of advances have been made, little can yet be done to avoid tamoxifen resistance. On the assumption that tamoxifen resistance may be related to metabolism of the drug to estrogenic compounds, several laboratories are looking at experimental drugs that are similar to tamoxifen in chemical structure but cannot be metabolized into estrogenic metabolites. Some of these, as well as other new agents, are showing promise against tamoxifen-resistant tumors.

7

**Tamoxifen for
Prevention in
Healthy Women**

The fight against breast cancer has recently taken a new turn. Disappointed by the lack of improved treatment over the past 20 years and fraught with concern about the possibility of developing the disease, many healthy women at high risk of developing breast cancer are choosing to participate in a controversial study. Its goal is to prevent these women from ever developing the disease—by means of tamoxifen, already commonly prescribed for the treatment of breast cancer. Although the drug is considered extremely safe in women with existing breast cancer, it does have a number of significant side effects (as discussed in Chapter 5). It is these side effects, and the unproved value of long-term administration of tamoxifen, that worry opponents of the study.

For many women, however, any action offers welcome relief from the chronic fear of breast cancer that has plagued them for years. The tamoxifen trial primarily recruits women who are considered at high risk of developing breast cancer. Many have a strong family history (mother, sister, daughter) of the disease, and the majority have watched the suffering and eventual death of

their relative. It is easy to understand why so many women are prepared to accept the risk of side effects from tamoxifen in order to avoid developing the cancer itself.

The concept of preventing the disease before it occurs appeals both to potential patients and to their doctors, who are often frustrated by their inability to help. Because breast cancer affects so many women and appears to be on the rise, powerful women's health groups have formed to make the public and the government aware of the significant suffering and loss of life from this disease (66).

WHAT IS THE TAMOXIFEN CHEMOPREVENTION TRIAL?

In an effort to address this overwhelming problem, the National Surgical Adjuvant Breast and Bowel Project (NSABP), headed by a number of renowned physicians, set out to design a study that would help prevent breast cancer. They reasoned that because in postmenopausal women the antiestrogenic agent tamoxifen is able to effectively prevent the recurrence of breast cancer in both the initially treated breast and in the "healthy" opposite breast, tamoxifen might also prevent the occurrence of breast cancer in women at high risk of developing the disease (47, 67–70). Tamoxifen had been used in the clinic for years and for an anticancer drug was considered relatively safe. The NSABP therefore decided to explore whether tamoxifen could prevent breast cancer in healthy women at high risk for developing the disease.

The 68-million-dollar study, primarily funded by the National Institutes of Health, started in 1992. By mid-1993 more than 8,000 healthy women were enrolled, out of a prospective 16,000. The NSABP predicts that tamoxifen will cause a 30 to 40 percent reduction in the incidence of breast cancer among these women. Proponents of the trial suggest that tamoxifen will have the added benefit of lowering the number of heart attacks and bone fractures of women taking the drug.

The goals of the study are to determine (1) whether tamoxifen therapy is effective in preventing invasive breast cancer in women

at increased risk for the disease, and (2) whether the mortality attributed to breast cancer is reduced by tamoxifen. In addition, the study will investigate whether tamoxifen lowers the incidence of fatal and nonfatal heart disease (myocardial infarction) and reduces the incidence of bone fractures.

WHY WAS THIS TRIAL INITIATED?

In the United States about 180,000 new cases of invasive breast cancer are diagnosed each year. Approximately one-third of these patients will eventually die of the disease (66). The incidence of breast cancer appears to be rising at a rate of 1 to 2 percent per year. The increase has been attributed primarily to the escalating longevity of elderly women, but it may also be influenced by improved detection techniques. Other risk factors, including the decision not to have children, the postponement of childbirth until after the age of 30, and potentially greater exposure to dietary or environmental hazards, may also be involved. The large number of women developing breast cancer (one in nine), and the lack of progress in treating the disease, emphasize the magnitude of the problem. While the avoidance of risk factors associated with the development of breast cancer is not always practical, the use of drugs to help prevent this disease (chemoprevention) may be a suitable option.

WHERE IS THE STUDY BEING PERFORMED?

The NSABP study is taking place at approximately 270 institutes across the country. The staff at each location is responsible for recruiting women for the study, for determination of eligibility, and for placement of eligible women in the study. Each institute will also be responsible for treatment of the patients enrolled and for final evaluation of the benefits.

In general, women entering are randomly assigned to one of two groups. Half will receive 20 mg of tamoxifen daily for five years, while the other half will receive a sugar-pill placebo. To avoid any

possible bias, patients will not know the group to which they have been assigned until the end of the study. During the trial each patient will be monitored closely by her physician to make certain that she is taking the drug regularly and evaluate whether she is experiencing any side effects. Blood sampling and other tests will be performed regularly to assess the effects of tamoxifen. Routine mammograms will be performed to establish if women in the tamoxifen group have a reduced rate of breast tumor occurrence, decreased mortality, or improved quality of life when compared to women in the placebo group.

WHAT RISK FACTORS ARE BEING CONSIDERED?

It is difficult to establish clearly many of the risk factors associated with breast cancer. Therefore, only those that have demonstrated significant association with the increased risk of breast cancer are being used to determine eligibility for the tamoxifen chemoprevention trial. These risk factors include:

1. The number of first-degree relatives (sister, mother, daughter) with breast cancer.
2. Whether or not the woman has had children.
3. Age at first live birth.
4. Number of breast biopsies performed to rule out breast cancer.
5. A diagnosis of atypical hyperplasia (abnormal proliferation of cells) upon biopsy.
6. Age at first menstrual period.
7. A diagnosis of lobular carcinoma in situ (LCIS) in women 35 or older.

HOW ARE THE RISK FACTORS DETERMINED FOR THE PREVENTION TRIAL?

For each woman in the trial the annual probability and the lifetime probability of developing breast cancer will be estimated by computer. The computer model used for these calculations is

known as the Gail risk model, originally designed with information generated by the Breast Cancer Detection Demonstration Project. The BCDDP studies routine annual mammographic screenings in women at increased risk for developing breast cancer and has the largest body of data available on such women.

In order to determine a woman's eligibility for the prevention trial, the physician plugs in the number of known risk factors she has that are associated with the development of breast cancer. A computer program then establishes the risk of developing breast cancer over the period of a year, or during the patient's lifetime, and compares it to the risk for a 60-year-old woman.

Because risk increases with age (see table 9), directors of the study have calculated minimum relative risks for eligibility at each

Table 9. *Incidence of Breast Cancer by Age, 1983 to 1987*

Age (years)	Average Annual Incidence (cases per 100,000)
35–39	66.1
40–44	126.5
45–49	186.6
50–54	221.1
55–59	272.1
60–64	334.8
65–69	392.3
70–74	417.8
75–79	443.9
80–84	442.1
85+	410.9

Source: Adapted from L. A. B. Ries, B. F. Hankey, and B. K. Edwards, eds. *Cancer Statistics Review, 1983–1987.* National Cancer Institute, Division of Cancer Prevention and Control Surveillance Program. National Institutes of Health Publ. No. 90-2789.

age. For instance, if you are 35 years old, the minimum relative risk required to enter the study is 5.07, which equals a 1.7 percent probability that you will develop breast cancer over a five-year period. If you are 55 years of age, the minimum relative risk to be eligible is only 1.23, which is also equal to a 1.7 percent probability of developing breast cancer over five years.

WHO CAN ENTER THE TRIAL?

All women over the age of 60 are eligible for the study. Women who are 35 to 59 years of age are evaluated for their eligibility based on the number or combination of risk factors they have that are associated with breast cancer. When a woman's combined risk factors are estimated to be equal to or greater than those of a 60-year-old woman, she is considered eligible to enter the study. The probability that a 60-year-old woman will develop breast cancer over a five-year period is 1.7 percent. Therefore, women younger than 60 must have at least an estimated 1.7 percent probability in order to enter into the trial. Women more than 35 years old with a diagnosis of LCIS are automatically considered for eligibility because this factor carries with it an almost tenfold increased risk of invasive breast cancer.

The study also accepts women on low-fat diets, lipid-lowering agents, anticoagulants, and other drugs for osteoporosis (biphosphonates, calcitonin, fluoride, vitamin D). Women at increased risk for osteoporosis from taking anticonvulsants, diuretics, or thyroid hormones may take part.

Thus, for each person interested in entering the study, the Gail model is used to estimate a composite relative risk of developing breast cancer. This figure is based on combining the risks for individual factors. The age-specific risks are then taken into account and a final breast cancer risk profile is developed and compared to that of a woman of the same age without added risk factors.

WHAT ARE MY CHANCES
OF ENTERING THE STUDY?

Obviously the more risk factors you have, the more likely you are to be eligible. Age appears to be the single most significant deter-

minant. About 0.3 percent of women who are 35 years old will have enough other risk factors to increase overall risk to the level required to enter the study; on the other hand, 12.5 percent of women 55 years of age are likely to be eligible.

For a woman 35 years of age, a history showing one or more first-degree relatives with breast cancer, and her own benign breast disease with at least two biopsies, would potentially make her eligible for the study. A 40-year-old patient may be entered solely on a history of first-degree relatives if two or more have the disease. She may also be eligible if she has had at least two biopsies for benign breast disease. By age 45 to 50, only one or more first-degree relatives with breast cancer, or benign breast disease with at least two breast biopsies, is required for eligibility to enter the trial.

WHO IS NOT ELIGIBLE FOR THE TAMOXIFEN CHEMOPREVENTION TRIAL?

Those who do not meet the eligibility criteria will be excluded from the trial. This group will include women between ages 35 and 60 who do not have significant risk factors for breast cancer and all women younger than 35 years of age.

A number of other factors will be considered. Women must have a life expectancy of at least ten years and no prior history of invasive breast cancer of any kind, including intraductal carcinoma in situ (DCIS) or previous lobular carcinoma in situ (LCIS) treated by mastectomy, radiation, or systemic adjuvant therapy. Women who have had any kind of cancer (except basal or squamous carcinoma of the skin or carcinoma in situ of the cervix) over the past ten years will not be eligible for the study. Women who have previously received tamoxifen will also be excluded.

Patients with existing nonmalignant disease that may result in their not being able to take tamoxifen will be barred from the study, as well as women whose activity is restricted for a significant portion of each day, who are pregnant, or who anticipate being pregnant while participating in the study. In addition, women with a history of deep-vein thrombosis or pulmonary embolism cannot be admitted. Those who have a psychiatric condition, including

history of clinical depression or addictive disorder that may interfere with their ability to knowingly consent to the study or take
medications regularly, will also be excluded.

Patients who are participating in other breast cancer prevention
trials involving the use of drugs will not be eligible for this study.
Nor will women currently taking oral contraceptives or estrogen or
progesterone therapy, unless the medications are stopped three
months prior to entering the tamoxifen study. Women with a prior
history of cardiovascular events (heart attacks) are eligible, pro-
vided their life expectancy is at least ten years.

WHAT IS REQUIRED TO ENTER THE STUDY?

Women who are interested in participating must first have their
breast cancer risk profile determined, including their age, family
history of breast cancer, number of breast biopsies and diagnosis,
and history of any live births. The family history of heart disease
and diabetes will be obtained. Other characteristics such as race,
residence, and education will be recorded. If a patient is found
eligible for the study, she will be asked to sign an informed consent
form that notifies her of potential risks or benefits of the study.

Women who are considered eligible will then undergo a detailed
evaluation of their medical history, with particular emphasis on
risk factors for breast cancer, cardiovascular disease, and osteoporosis. A full family history of breast and cardiovascular disease
will also be obtained. The requisite physical examination will include breast exam, gynecologic exam, mammogram, blood pres-
sure, weight, and height. Laboratory tests will also be performed to
determine blood count, cholesterol level, and liver and kidney
function. An electrocardiogram will be taken in patients 55 years
of age or older.

WHAT DO I DO ONCE I'M A PARTICIPANT?

When a woman is found eligible for the study and has undergone
the preliminary evaluation, she is assigned to one of two groups.
Members of one group will receive two tamoxifen tablets (10 mg

each) that must be taken once a day for at least five years. Members of the other unit will receive a placebo tablet that cannot be distinguished from tamoxifen. The patient will not know which group she is in until the study evaluation is complete.

Participants will be asked to come to the center for routine follow-ups. The first such exams will be three and six months after the beginning of the study, then every six months for the remaining five years. If a patient remains on tamoxifen beyond five years, she will be followed on a yearly basis.

The examinations will consist of an update of the medical history, with special emphasis on potential side effects of tamoxifen —any illnesses, hospitalizations, operations, or fractures. The breasts will be examined at each visit, and any suspicious lumps will be biopsied. Laboratory tests and physical exams will be performed at each follow-up visit, with annual mammograms and gynecologic exams. Participants will be asked about any side effects of the drug, including menstrual irregularities and visual changes.

For the first three months of the study, each participant will be contacted monthly to ensure that she is taking the pills as directed. And she will be asked to assess how well she has done with regard to taking the pills regularly.

WHAT HAPPENS IF I DEVELOP BREAST CANCER WHILE ON THE STUDY?

Tamoxifen therapy is intended to prevent the occurrence of breast cancer and is expected to reduce the incidence of breast cancer in patients in the tamoxifen treatment group. If, however, tamoxifen is not as effective as the individuals who developed the trial anticipate, or if by chance it even stimulates tumor growth, as others have suggested, then a number of women may develop tumors during the study. If so, they will not necessarily be removed from the trial.

Patients who develop tumors that are considered noninvasive, such as LCIS or DCIS, may continue in the tamoxifen study as planned. The physician may use local methods of controlling the cancer, such as lumpectomy, surgery, or radiation; but the pres-

ence or absence of tamoxifen seems to have little effect on these other cancers.

The detection of invasive breast cancer is, however, a reason to remove patients from the study. Women who develop invasive breast cancer while on tamoxifen will be evaluated carefully, and the appropriate therapy will be given for the type of cancer present. Typically any new breast cancer will be evaluated for the presence of estrogen and progesterone receptors, and patients with estrogen-receptor-positive breast cancer will be placed on a tamoxifen regimen. However, if a participant has an estrogen-receptor-positive tumor that has developed while she is already taking tamoxifen, it must be assumed that she is resistant to tamoxifen; she will not be given additional tamoxifen therapy, as would most patients with estrogen-receptor-positive breast cancer. But if the patient developed a tumor while taking the placebo tablets and she is diagnosed with a form of cancer that will respond to tamoxifen, her physician may place her on tamoxifen.

CAN I BE TAKEN OFF THE STUDY
FOR OTHER REASONS?

The diagnosis of other nonbreast forms of cancer (except for basal or squamous cell carcinoma of the skin or carcinoma in situ of the cervix) will be sufficient reason for removal from the study. Women who develop and are diagnosed with pulmonary embolism or deep-vein thrombosis may also be withdrawn. Those who become pregnant during the study will be discontinued until the completion or termination of the pregnancy or breast feeding. Patients who develop significant depression while participating may be asked to discontinue tamoxifen, but may resume taking it when the depression has resolved. In addition, individuals who develop any serious side effects of tamoxifen, including visual problems (retinal changes, corneal scarring), will no longer take part.

WHAT IS EXPECTED TO COME
OUT OF THIS STUDY?

The primary emphasis of the study is on whether tamoxifen can decrease the incidence and mortality of invasive breast cancer. The

study investigators believe that a 30 to 40 percent reduction in breast cancer incidence is feasible. The secondary goals are to evaluate whether tamoxifen decreases the occurrence of and mortality of women from heart disease. The researchers suggest that there may be a reduction as high as 56 percent in coronary heart disease, and a 38 percent reduction in myocardial infarction from the use of tamoxifen for five years. Finally, the study hopes to determine if there is a difference in the fracture rate of women receiving tamoxifen and those in the placebo group. The estimate is that a 57 percent reduction in hip fractures will be noted in women taking tamoxifen.

CAN I GET MY DOCTOR TO PRESCRIBE TAMOXIFEN FOR ME?

Tamoxifen has been on the market for some time, but only for use in the treatment of breast cancer patients. In this group of patients it has already been tested and the benefits have been carefully weighed against the risks. Unfortunately, since the conception of this study a number of nonparticipating physicians have prescribed tamoxifen to healthy women who are considered at high risk of developing the disease. Because the use of tamoxifen in this subset of patients has been proved neither safe nor effective, these physicians are putting their patients at risk by offering the drug to them. While most side effects are considered minimal in breast cancer patients, several life-threatening side effects must be closely monitored by a doctor who is familiar with the drug. In addition, there are those who feel that the drug should not be given to healthy women (see Chapter 8 for their arguments). Furthermore, it is considered unacceptable medical practice to prescribe drugs for non-FDA-approved medicinal uses.

8

The Ongoing Controversy over the Tamoxifen Chemoprevention Trial

Few would dispute that the prevention of breast cancer is one of the most important areas of cancer research today. With the extraordinary percentage of women developing the disease and the slow advances in successful treatment, prevention is the most sensible goal. Advocates of the tamoxifen trial clearly understand the need for studies addressing the prevention of breast cancer and feel that tamoxifen is well suited for this purpose.

On the other side of the issue stand a number of physicians and scientists, and several women's groups, who are strongly opposed to the tamoxifen trial. Although they acknowledge that the study is well intentioned, they fear that implementation is premature and that the design lacks sufficient scientific merit. They suggest that there is little evidence to support the notion that tamoxifen is more beneficial than harmful when given to healthy women. They point to the numerous side effects of tamoxifen, including hot flashes, menstrual irregularities, eye problems, secondary cancers, and fatal blood clots in a small proportion of patients. They argue that these may be acceptable risks in a population known to have breast

cancer, in that the benefits from tamoxifen generally outweigh the liabilities, but that the risks may be unacceptable in healthy women. Critics further suggest that the secondary benefits relative to cardiovascular disease and osteoporosis are overestimated, and that the small amount of projected gain to women in the trial is not worth the risk involved.

WHAT ARE THE PROJECTED
BENEFITS AND RISKS?

The directors of the study have projected that of the 8,000 women in the trial taking tamoxifen, 124 are likely to develop breast cancer. Of the 8,000 women taking no drug (receiving the placebo), 186 (1.7 percent) are likely to develop breast cancer while participating in the study (71). Therefore the net projected benefit is that 62 women may be prevented from developing breast cancer, or one woman for every four cancer centers involved in the study.

Critics suggest that even though 62 women may avoid breast cancer, all 8,000 women taking tamoxifen will be subjected to its side effects, some of which are life threatening. Of those women, opponents of the study project that 1,300 will experience hot flashes, 1,136 will have vaginal discharges, 480 will have irregular menses, 272 will develop skin rashes, 56 will develop thrombocytopenia, between 31 and 53 will develop uterine (endometrial) tumors, 16 will experience mild inflammation of the veins (superficial phlebitis), 24 will have moderate inflammation of the veins, 24 will undergo deep venous thrombosis (blood clots in the large veins) requiring hospitalization, and another 24 will develop life-threatening pulmonary emboli (blood clots in the lungs). There is the further potential for a number of deaths from tamoxifen-related side effects, primarily associated with thromboembolic disease. It is a matter of opinion whether the prevention of breast cancer in 62 women, many of whom would be completely curable by standard treatment, is worth putting healthy women at risk of unpleasant or even potentially life-threatening side effects.

We must also remember that the projected benefits and risks from this study were primarily derived from research on breast

cancer patients given tamoxifen twice a day for five years. In these studies tamoxifen was shown to prevent the recurrence of cancer in the contralateral breast in postmenopausal women (47, 67–69). The evidence also suggested that patients who took tamoxifen survived longer than those who did not.

Critics of the present study point out that while tamoxifen may effectively prevent recurrence or new cancers in the contralateral breast of postmenopausal women with known breast cancer, these results cannot accurately predict the benefits in the breast tissue of healthy women. The comparison may be flawed in that the "healthy" breast of the women studied may already be genetically predisposed to the development of breast cancer because of the disease in the other breast. The vast majority of tumors that arise in the remaining healthy breast are in fact new tumors. Therefore, the benefits of tamoxifen in the contralateral breast of women with prior breast cancer may overestimate the benefits to women who are only at high risk for developing the disease.

In an article critical of the tamoxifen study, Dr. Adriane Fugh-Berman and Dr. Samuel Epstein report that the drug may act by suppressing the growth in the healthy breast of cancer cells that are similar in nature to those found in the diseased breast. Tamoxifen may not prevent the growth of new tumors that differ in their characteristics from the original tumor. Moreover, these authors state that "both breasts of a woman with breast cancer have been exposed to identical genetic, reproductive, hormonal, and environmental influences, and that there is no scientific basis for regarding the contralateral breast of a woman with breast cancer as a 'healthy control'" (6, pp. 340–341).

Although tamoxifen is extremely effective in preventing disease recurrence in women who have had the disease, we still cannot accurately predict which healthy patients are genetically prone to develop breast cancer, and which may benefit from tamoxifen chemoprevention. The risks of taking tamoxifen are well known and must be carefully weighed against the potential gain a healthy woman might derive from taking the drug. One recently published analysis concluded that "for healthy women, the NSABP

trial is as likely to prove tamoxifen a net detriment as a benefit" (35, p. 233).

CAN WE ACCURATELY PREDICT WHICH WOMEN ARE AT HIGH RISK OF DEVELOPING BREAST CANCER?

The known risk factors associated with the development of breast cancer are still considered ambiguous. We have said previously that only one-third of women with breast cancer have any of the known risk factors that are evaluated for admittance into the tamoxifen study (6). Of the one-third who do, most share the major risk factors of age (50 years or older) and strong family history of the disease (mother, daughter, or sister with breast cancer, particularly when premenopausal).

WHO SHOULD BE CONSIDERED AT HIGH RISK?

Advocates of the study suggest that all women over the age of 60 should be considered at high risk of developing breast cancer, and all should be eligible for the trial. Because these women are post-menopausal, proponents also believe that these women would benefit from the potential protective effects of tamoxifen on both heart and bone. Additionally, it is in this age group that tamoxifen has been shown to effectively prevent further cancer in the contra-lateral breast of women with previous cancer in one breast.

SHOULD PREMENOPAUSAL PATIENTS BE ELIGIBLE FOR THE STUDY?

Premenopausal patients who are considered at high risk of developing the disease are being accepted for the study. Proponents suggest that this is the best time to intervene in disease prevention, for the risk rises significantly with age in the postmenopausal years. At least one review has suggested that tamoxifen may have a

beneficial effect in premenopausal women with estrogen-receptor-positive breast cancer (72).

Critics of the tamoxifen trial express scientific concern over the eligibility of premenopausal women and suggest that these patients may receive limited benefit from tamoxifen. They point to evidence presented by the Cancer Research Campaign Breast Cancer Trials Group, which indicates that while tamoxifen may reduce the risk of contralateral breast cancer in postmenopausal patients, it actually increases the risk of contralateral breast cancer in premenopausal patients years after tamoxifen therapy is stopped (73). Although it is not clearly established, premenopausal women might also be at increased risk of developing tamoxifen-induced uterine cancers (32–34). In similar trials under way in Britain and Italy, only women aged 45 to 65 who have had hysterectomies are allowed to take part in tamoxifen chemoprevention trials. Premenopausal women without hysterectomies are excluded primarily because of the previous data attributing the increased incidence of endometrial cancer to tamoxifen.

Another adverse factor is that even if tamoxifen is effective in preventing contralateral breast cancer in premenopausal patients with estrogen-receptor-positive breast cancer, the majority of premenopausal women who develop breast cancer have estrogen-receptor-negative breast tumors that are considered much less responsive to tamoxifen (6). Since estrogen-receptor-negative premenopausal patients are typically excluded from studies of tamoxifen, there are no data defining the role of tamoxifen in preventing contralateral breast cancer in these women.

IS TAMOXIFEN SAFE WHEN GIVEN LONG TERM?

There is little information on the use of tamoxifen for more than ten years, even in women with breast cancer. Critics therefore oppose the inclusion of healthy women, even those with increased risk of developing breast cancer (greater than 1.7 percent), to study the side effects of long-term tamoxifen therapy. Further-

more, because the potential benefit from tamoxifen probably only occurs while the drug is being taken, women might need to take tamoxifen for the rest of their lives—a decision that obviously would have unknown results. At least one toxicity has already been associated with cumulative dosing of tamoxifen: both reversible and irreversible eye damage has been demonstrated after prolonged use (54, 74). At this time we do not know what other side effects may emerge with longer-term dosing of tamoxifen. Other toxicities, such as liver cancer, have been noted with long-term tamoxifen use in laboratory animals (75, 76). While there is little evidence that liver cancer is associated with tamoxifen use in humans, critics of the prevention study claim that submitting healthy women to even the slightest risk of drug-induced liver cancer is not acceptable.

COULD TAMOXIFEN HAVE OTHER ADVERSE EFFECTS IN WOMEN CONSIDERED AT HIGH RISK FOR DEVELOPING THE DISEASE?

For years laboratory researchers have been obtaining some very puzzling findings. While tamoxifen is commonly considered a drug that inhibits or slows the growth of cancer cells, it has also been reported to stimulate tumor growth in animals. In the vast majority of cases where estrogen receptors are present in cancer cells, tamoxifen inhibits growth. Under certain conditions, however, both estrogen-receptor-negative and estrogen-receptor-positive cells have been found to grow in the presence of tamoxifen (75, 77, 78).

Opponents of the tamoxifen trial interpret these results to mean that if a woman is genetically predisposed to get the disease, or has a small number of breast cancer cells that have not yet grown to detectable size, exposure to tamoxifen may have an adverse effect. They suggest that the cancer cells may learn to tolerate tamoxifen, and potentially even be stimulated to grow in its presence. They argue that when and if such breast cancer cells do grow, they will be much more aggressive than the usual breast cancer cells.

Studies done in rodents demonstrate that tamoxifen reduces the incidence of breast cancer induced by cancer-causing chemicals; but when tumors do develop, they are a highly aggressive variety that spreads rapidly (78, 79).

COULD TAMOXIFEN STIMULATE THE GROWTH OF TUMORS IN BREAST CANCER PATIENTS?

Fortunately for most patients with estrogen-receptor-positive breast cancer who are taking tamoxifen, their breast tumors are responsive to the drug, and it acts to inhibit the growth of breast cancer. But even after an initial positive response, tamoxifen therapy becomes ineffective in many patients. Their tumors may in fact become somewhat dependent on tamoxifen for growth, as evidenced by the fact that tumor responses (stabilization or regression) have been noted in some women after merely discontinuing the drug (64, 65, 80).

WILL TAMOXIFEN WORK FOR A LONG PERIOD?

Critics of the study also note that while many patients who have breast cancer initially derive significant benefits from tamoxifen, virtually all patients at some point stop responding to the drug and their tumors recur. The development of tamoxifen resistance typically takes place after about two years (20, 59). The reasons why the tumor cells stop responding are unknown. Those opposed to the study therefore suggest that tamoxifen's preventive effects are most likely of short duration despite the strong early benefit (81). Moreover, if a patient develops breast cancer while taking tamoxifen, she might also be resistant to one of the primary agents used in treatment. Or she might be predisposed to develop a type of breast cancer that lacks estrogen receptors, which is generally a more aggressive variety (82).

WHAT ABOUT THE CLAIMS THAT TAMOXIFEN WILL ALSO PREVENT HEART DISEASE AND OSTEOPOROSIS?

To date only a few clinical studies have addressed the potential benefits of tamoxifen in preventing either heart disease or osteoporosis, and those that have show varying results. Critics suggest that the claims at the very least are premature, if not overly optimistic.

Will Tamoxifen Decrease the Risk of Heart Attack?   In women more than 60 years old, the risk of heart attack rises substantially with age. This is also true of men. In addition, there is a linear increase in the risk of heart disease in men when total cholesterol levels exceed 200 mg percent (6). This relationship is seen in women, but only when levels reach 270 mg percent. More important, in women the risk of heart disease appears to be related more to the type of cholesterol than to the total cholesterol level. Low levels of the "good" cholesterol (high-density lipoprotein, or HDL) appear to be a more accurate indicator of heart disease than high levels of "bad" cholesterol (low-density lipoprotein, or LDL; 83).

In postmenopausal women the use of conjugated estrogens has been shown to consistently decrease LDL and increase HDL (84). These effects may significantly lower the incidence of heart disease in women. Because tamoxifen has been noted to have some estrogenic effects on cholesterol levels, it was at one time assumed that it may have the same favorable effects in the prevention of heart disease. To date there is little convincing evidence in support of this assumption, however.

Clinical studies have yielded conflicting information about tamoxifen and cholesterol levels (85). Although tamoxifen has been reported in most studies to decrease total cholesterol levels, other reports have suggested that it can increase these levels—perhaps even strikingly (86, 87). Its effects on concentrations of "good" cholesterol are still more ambiguous. Tamoxifen's effects on "bad" cholesterol appear more consistent, with reports showing a de-

crease in LDL on the order of 20 percent (88). But high levels of LDL do not appear to be as reliable an indicator of heart disease in women as in men (83).

At present the net effect of tamoxifen on cholesterol level and its role in the prevention of heart disease are debatable. Encouraging results from a Scottish group suggest that tamoxifen may decrease the mortality from coronary heart disease (89). Still, of eight randomized trials of tamoxifen in breast cancer patients this was the only study to report such a decrease. To date clinical evidence fails to substantiate a favorable role of tamoxifen in preventing heart disease.

Does Tamoxifen Prevent Osteoporosis?   The loss of bone mineral density is significantly influenced by hormonal changes. Following menopause most women are placed on estrogen replacement therapy to maintain significant levels of estrogen in the hope of preventing osteoporosis and its associated bone fractures. Most postmenopausal patients who have been diagnosed with breast cancer, however, particularly those who have estrogen-receptor-positive breast cancers, are not given estrogen replacement therapy owing to the increased likelihood of breast cancer recurrence. The risk of osteoporosis in this group remains a significant problem.

Tamoxifen is considered an antiestrogen, so at one time it was believed that tamoxifen given postmenopausally might increase the risk of osteoporosis. But several animal and human studies performed in postmenopausal patients suggest that tamoxifen may act like estrogen in preserving bone mineral density (90–92). In a small clinical study giving tamoxifen (10 mg twice daily) for two years, the drug was shown to prevent decreases in the bone density of the lower back (lumbar spine) and to have no apparent adverse effects on radial bone density (bones in the forearm; 93–95). The unknown effects of tamoxifen on the pelvic bones and the bones in the hip are perhaps much more important, because hip fractures account for the majority of hospitalizations resulting from osteoporosis (6). The effects on bone density of using tamoxifen for more than five years also are unclear, especially in premenopausal patients.

WHAT WERE THE RESULTS OF
CONGRESSIONAL HEARINGS
ON THE STUDY?

In testimony before several congressional subcommittees formed in October 1992 to review the safety of the tamoxifen trial, opponents expressed their concerns about both the design of the research and the ethics of performing such a study in healthy women. After the first round of hearings, anxiety was expressed over the informed-consent process which is intended to notify patients of potential hazards. Both state and federal law requires that participants completely understand all risks involved in a given study, and sign a consent form acknowledging that they fully comprehend those risks. There were complaints that many of the medical centers involved in the tamoxifen trial utilized consent forms that did not adequately inform women of all the potential risks that they might encounter.

After reviewing the information on the consent forms, members of the congressional staff found that, in general, the potential benefits to the study were presented in an overly optimistic way and crucial information concerning the risks was lacking. They noted that in 62 percent of the centers conducting the study, information on the patient consent forms concerning the risk of blood clots was either misleading or nonexistent. When this risk was described, many of the consent forms merely mentioned that the prediction was for three instances of blood clots. Yet this particular side effect is known to occur in 1.5 percent of women taking tamoxifen and is a potentially life-threatening event (38, 47, 96). Thus, of the 8,000 women taking tamoxifen, 48 are expected to experience some degree of clotting and as many as 8 to 21 women may develop fatal blood clots.

During the congressional hearings it became evident that those testifying felt there was a tendency of the medical community to downplay the side effects of tamoxifen. When the side effects of other anticancer agents are compared, tamoxifen does seem a rather benign drug; however, as one woman who had been treated with tamoxifen testified, "While the side effects were

not life threatening, they certainly threatened the quality of my life."

After hearing hours of testimony, the chair of the hearings, Rep. Donald M. Payne (D-N.J.), expressed his concern about new data that had emerged since the start of the study. He cited a 1992 report from the Royal Marsden Hospital in London (73). In it tamoxifen was shown to effectively prevent the recurrence of breast cancer in postmenopausal women; but in the group of premenopausal patients taking tamoxifen, the incidence of breast cancer was greater than expected.

Earlier, in July 1991 a Food and Drug Administration (FDA) advisory committee evaluating the tamoxifen study separately had recommended that premenopausal women not be admitted. The National Cancer Institute felt that this restriction would significantly limit the number of individuals recruited to the study and make it difficult to achieve the desired enrollment of 16,000 women. Although the FDA finally allowed the study to proceed as planned, many of the FDA committee members remained opposed to the inclusion of premenopausal women (75).

THE TRIAL GOES ON

Despite criticism, congressional review, and the many hurdles involved in initiating such a controversial study, the tamoxifen trial has proceeded resolutely and has already recruited more than 8,000 healthy women. As such women continue to sign up for the study, its supporters and opponents continue their war of words in the health columns of many local newspapers. Critics attack primarily the inclusion of premenopausal women, claiming that there is now enough scientific evidence to suggest that tamoxifen may put these patients at an even higher risk of developing breast cancer. Investigators involved in the study defend their inclusion of these women and suggest that all groundbreaking research has questions and risks. They deemphasize the side effects of tamoxifen and state that it is not an experimental drug but a widely used breast cancer agent that has been thoroughly studied over a long period. As for tamoxifen's more serious toxicities, the researchers

say that they exclude women who might be expected to have severe side effects and that they believe that close monitoring of patients should alleviate most of the remaining problems.

Caught between the arguments are the women already participating in the study and those considering enrollment. Frustrated with the lack of choices, they are willing to enter the trial regardless of the potential side effects they may encounter. Partially out of fear and partially out of desire to help others down the road, these women march forward bravely while doctors and scientists on both sides eagerly await the results.

9

Future Approaches

Owing to the rather slow progress in the treatment of breast cancer, there is a movement toward early detection and prevention of the disease. Trials focusing on dietary measures, drug therapy, prophylactic mastectomies, and routine mammography are currently under way.

CAN A LOW-FAT DIET
PREVENT BREAST CANCER?

Because a diet high in fat appears to be a risk factor in the development of breast cancer, reduced dietary fats may be important to prevention of the disease. The Women's Health Initiative is one group that is investigating diet and its relation to breast cancer development. The study, which began in 1993, will explore over a ten-year period whether a diet low in fat and high in fruits and vegetables will reduce the incidence of breast cancer in postmenopausal women. The use of estrogen replacement in postmenopausal patients to prevent osteoporosis and heart disease will also be evaluated. Approximately 70,000 women will participate. Each will be randomly assigned to go on the diet, take estrogen replacement, or both. In view of the dearth of data on the benefits of estrogen replacement in these diseases, and the slightly increased risk of developing breast cancer and endometrial cancer from estrogen, these studies are expected to advance our knowledge substantially.

WHAT ABOUT HORMONAL AGENTS?

Many forms of breast cancer are hormone responsive, and the survival of hormone-sensitive tumors is dependent on estrogen. So the use of hormones that counter estrogen action would seem a feasible means to prevent breast cancer.

The use of synthesized or "exogenous" hormones to prevent cancer is not a new idea. It has long been known that the low doses of estrogen and progesterone found in birth control pills may provide some protection against cancers of the ovary and uterus. In these types of cancer the use of birth control pills has actually reduced the incidence of disease and the mortality rate.

Birth control pills have had little effect in controlling breast cancer, however. Because some forms are highly dependent on estrogen for growth, this fact is not surprising. As discussed in a recent article in *Science* (97), the incidence of breast cancer rises sharply with age during the premenopausal years; thus it is this population that appears best suited for hormonal intervention to prevent breast cancer.

At least one study already targets premenopausal women with a form of hormone therapy that will act both as birth control and as chemoprevention for breast cancer (98). Hormones called gonadotropin-releasing hormone agonists (GNRHAs) are given to premenopausal women. These hormones inhibit ovulation and reduce the number of hormones that are naturally synthesized by the ovary. Their action includes reducing the amount of estrogen secreted by the ovaries to levels that approach those of the postmenopausal period. Small amounts of estrogen or progesterone can then be added back, to avoid side effects similar to those seen in menopause.

The goal of this study is to provide an effective contraceptive agent in premenopausal women that will reduce both ovarian and uterine cancer risk as well as prevent breast cancer. The anticipated benefits are estimated to be quite high: a 31 percent reduction in the incidence of breast cancer over a women's lifetime if the contraceptive is used for five years, 47 percent if used for ten years, and 70 percent if used for fifteen years. The protection against ovarian cancer (41 percent if used for five years) is expected to be very similar to that seen with combination oral contraceptives (COCs). The reduction in endometrial cancer is expected to be somewhat less than that afforded by COCs (18 percent compared to 46 percent from COCs used for five years; 97, 98).

CAN NEW DRUGS BE MADE TO BLOCK THE ESTROGEN RECEPTORS?

The further evaluation of how tamoxifen inhibits breast cancer cell growth has pointed out our limited knowledge of how this drug really works. Although tamoxifen does bind to estrogen receptors to block the effects of estrogens, this binding ability of tamoxifen and other antiestrogenic agents does not correlate perfectly with how well it inhibits tumor cell growth. The poor correlation has been frustrating for the development of new drugs; it means that binding of the drug to estrogen receptors and blockage of estrogen on the receptors cannot be used as tests to determine if a related agent is useful. Many scientists believe that tamoxifen may in fact produce effects on the cell that are unrelated to the estrogen receptor.

CAN BIOLOGICAL THERAPIES BE USED TO PREVENT BREAST CANCER?

We have only begun to understand the complex role of biological factors associated with the development of breast cancer. Much of what we do know is centered on the estrogen and progesterone receptors found in breast cancer cells that are hormonally sensitive. The presence or absence of these receptors has helped us to identify which patients will respond to antiestrogen therapy and, in some cases, what their chances of survival will be. Patients who have tumors that contain these hormone receptors tend to have a better overall survival rate than those who do not. While this information has helped us in the diagnosis, treatment, and prognosis of patients, to date hormone receptor status has not aided us in the prevention of breast cancer.

More recent studies have identified in breast cancer cells a number of new proteins that may be involved in the development of cancer. Several "families" have been identified. Many of these proteins are referred to as growth factors, because they actually stimulate the growth of cells. Secreted by cancer cells or other types of cells, they can act on proteins on the surface of breast cancer cells to stimulate cell growth. The proteins found on the surface of breast cancer cells are referred to as growth factor receptors. Additional proteins have been identified that may be associated with the potential of breast cancer cells to metastasize or spread from one area to another.

Ongoing studies of the proteins associated with breast cancer may lead to improved diagnosis, further prognostic information, and perhaps specific treatment regimens for individual patients. For example, biological agents such as monoclonal antibodies (immune factors that can be directed against specific proteins) can potentially be made that will block the receptors on the surface of breast cancer cells, thus preventing the growth factors from stimulating the tumor cells. Antibodies can also be attached to certain types of chemotherapy drugs so that the antibodies act like guided missiles delivering the toxic drug directly to the breast cancer cells. Other agents are being developed to bind directly to the growth factors and sequester them before they can stimulate the tumor cells to grow and divide (99).

Further studies will undoubtedly supply us with a wealth of information about the biology of breast cancer, and potentially about the defect present in breast cells that makes some women susceptible to getting the disease. Although biological agents have not had great success in the treatment of breast cancer, the future may hold more promise for these types of agents.

WHAT ABOUT PROPHYLACTIC MASTECTOMIES?

The idea of surgically removing the breasts to avoid breast cancer seems an exceedingly unattractive option to many women. Yet others feel it may relieve them of the chronic worry of developing breast cancer. This option is obviously restricted to those in a very high risk group for developing breast cancer (women with two or more first-degree relatives who have died of the disease, women whose biopsies are abnormal but not yet cancerous, or women who have had numerous breast biopsies leaving them severely scarred). Unfortunately, we still have only limited ability to define who is at risk for developing breast cancer, and what combination of factors puts a woman at truly high risk. Perhaps with improvements in the ability to detect seriously high risk, this type of preventive therapy will become more useful.

Furthermore, information on the true benefits of this procedure is sparse. It is often difficult to distinguish breast tissue from the surrounding tissues, and if even 5 percent of breast tissue remains after surgery, there is still a chance of developing breast cancer. At least a handful of patients have gone on to develop breast cancer despite preventive surgical mastectomy. It is extremely important that women understand the limitations of the procedure, especially that it provides no assurance that they will not go on to develop breast cancer anyway.

DON'T ROUTINE MAMMOGRAMS CATCH BREAST CANCER EARLY ENOUGH TO PREVENT ITS SPREAD?

Routine mammograms are very useful in detecting breast cancers before they have a chance to grow locally or spread to other parts of the body. They are not 100 percent accurate, however, and depend on the radiologist's ability to obtain a definitive X-ray. The test in very young women is considered less accurate than when they are older, primarily because of the higher density of tissues earlier in life. Most physicians suggest that a baseline mammogram be performed between the ages of 35 and 40, followed by a yearly examination. The test is also somewhat less accurate in women who have either very large or very small breasts. Therefore, regular physical examinations by a doctor and monthly self-examinations should always be performed in addition to mammography.

CONCLUSION

Although these approaches to early detection and prevention of breast cancer must still be proved effective, they may eventually play an integral role in reducing the incidence of several women's diseases. To date, it appears that routine mammography after the age of 35, a low-fat diet coupled with physical activity, and acceptable preventive measures may circumvent breast cancer, heart disease, and possibly osteoporosis (5, 100).

Glossary

Agonist   A drug that produces a response.

Antagonist   A drug that prevents the action of an agonist by acting on its specific receptor, or site.

Antiestrogen   A drug that blocks the effects of estrogen.

Aspirate   To remove by suction, using a syringe or other device.

Axillary   Pertaining to or situated near the axilla (armpit).

Calcification   The deposition of calcium salts within tissues.

Cell division   The process whereby a cell copies its genetic material (DNA) and then divides to maintain the exact amount of genetic material found in the original cell. The way in which cells multiply.

Chemoprevention   The inhibition of development, activation, or spread of a disease by administration of a chemical agent.

Chemotherapy   In general, the treatment of disease with chemical compounds or drugs. In the context of this book, the use of cytotoxins for treatment of breast cancer.

Chemotherapy cycles   The repeated administration of cytotoxic chemotherapy on a scheduled basis, usually every three to four weeks.

Cyst   A cavity or sac lined with abnormal tissue that usually contains fluid or other material.

Cytoplasm   The part of the cell that surrounds the nucleus, where the genetic material is stored.

Cytostatic   Capable of inhibiting the growth and multiplication of cells.

Cytotoxic   Having the effect of poisoning or destroying cells.

Disease-free survival   The time a patient remains free of disease, subsequent to initial treatment.

DNA (deoxyribonucleic acid)   The primary genetic material found in chromosomes, which holds all the information that the cell requires for growth and multiplication.

Ducts   Channels that transport such substances as the milk in breast tissue.

Estrogen   A steroid hormone made and secreted by the ovaries; involved in the menstrual cycle and in the growth and maturation of female secondary sex characteristics.

Estrogen receptors   Specific proteins, found within cells, that bind estrogen to produce a biological response (such as stimulation of cell growth).

Fibrocystic disease   A disease of the breast in which women have recurrent cysts containing both fibrous and cystic components.

Haploidy   The condition of having only a single set of chromosomes in a cell. Humans normally contain 46 chromosomes per cell; however, cancer cells and some others may become haploid and have only 23 chromosomes.

Hormone   A substance secreted by specialized cells of the endocrine glands (such as estrogen from the ovary).

Hyperplasia   An increase in the number of cells in a tissue or organ with a concomitant increase in the size of the structure involved.

Lymph nodes   The portion of the lymphatic system that functions to drain fluids from all parts of the body; situated along the lymph vessels.

Mammography   Radiographic (X-ray) examination of the breast.

Metabolize   To subject to metabolic change; to break down (chemically) a drug or foodstuff for utilization or removal from the body.

Metastasis   The transfer of a disease from one body site to another (specifically, the secondary growth of a malignant tumor at a site separate from the primary site from which it derived).

Nucleus   A membrane-bounded compartment of the cell that contains the genetic material DNA.

Overall survival   The length of time a patient survives following initial treatment.

Pathology   Study of the structural and functional changes associated with the disease process.

Perimenopausal   Referring to the period (approximately three years) when symptoms of menopause appear but menstruation continues.

Postmenopausal   Pertaining to the time after a woman has experienced menopause and is no longer menstruating.

Premenopausal   Occurring prior to menopause.

Progesterone   A hormone, secreted by the unfertilized egg, that is involved in the regulation of menstruation.

Replication   The cellular process of producing multiple copies of a molecule (such as DNA), each copy being identical with the original.

RNA (ribonucleic acid)   A substance found in the cell nucleus that consists of long copies of DNA. From the DNA it carries the genetic information that eventually will be processed into protein.

S-phase   The portion of the cell cycle in which DNA is replicated before it divides, so that the cell appears to have two copies of the DNA.

Synergistic   Having the capacity to act together so that the combined action of two or more substances is more effective than the action of any one acting individually.

Synthetic   Artificially produced by chemical procedure rather than obtained from a natural source.

Systemic   Relating to the whole system.

Systemic chemotherapy   Delivery of chemotherapy to the entire body, usually via the blood.

Toxin   A substance that is poisonous to cells and organisms.

Transcription   The process by which RNA is made from DNA.

Translation   The process by which specific proteins are made from RNA.

References

1. Harris, J. R., Morrow, M., and Bonadonna, G. Cancer of the breast. In *Cancer: Principles and Practice of Oncology*, V. T. DeVita, S. Hellman, and S. A. Rosenberg, eds. Philadelphia: J. B. Lippincott, 1993 (4th ed.), 1264–1332.

2. Merkle, D. E., and McGuire, W. L. Ploidy proliferative activity and prognosis: DNA flow cytometry of solid tumors. *Cancer* 65: 1194–1206 (1990).

3. Rose, D. P. Dietary fiber, phytoestrogens, and breast cancer. *Nutrition* 8: 47 (1992).

4. Carroll, K. K. Experimental evidence of dietary factors and hormone dependent cancers. *Cancer Res.* 35: 3374 (1975).

5. Wynder, E. L., Fujita, Y., Harris, R. E., Hirayama, T., and Hiyama, T. Comparative epidemiology of cancer between the United States and Japan. *Cancer* 67: 746 (1991).

6. Fugh-Berman, A., and Epstein, S. Tamoxifen: Disease prevention or disease substitution. *Lancet* 2: 340 (1992).

7. Buzdar, A. U. Adjuvant therapy for breast cancer. *Adv. Oncol.* 8: 10 (1992).

8. Bonadonna, G., Valagussa, P., Zembetti, M., Buzzoni, R., and

Moliterni, A. Milan adjuvant trials for stages I–II breast cancer. In *Adjuvant Therapy of Cancer,* S. E. Salmon, ed. Orlando, Fla.: Grune and Stratton, 1987, 211–221.

9. Buzzoni, R., Bonadonna, G., Valagussa, P., and Zambetti, M. Adjuvant chemotherapy with doxorubicin plus cyclophosphamide, methotrexate and fluorouracil in treatment of resectable breast cancer with more than three positive axillary nodes. *J. Clin. Oncol.* 9: 2136 (1991).

10. Ang, P. T., Buzdar, A. U., Smith, T. L., Kau, S., and Hortobagyi, G. N. Analysis of dose intensity in doxorubicin-containing adjuvant chemotherapy in stages II and III breast carcinoma. *J. Clin. Oncol.* 7: 1677 (1989).

11. Legha, S. S. Tamoxifen in the treatment of breast cancer. *Ann. Int. Med.* 1: 219 (1988).

12. Emmens, C. W. Postcoital contraception. *Brit. Med. Bull.* 26: 45 (1970).

13. Lunan, C. B., and Liopper, A. Antiestrogens: A review. *Clin. Endocrin.* 4: 551 (1975).

14. Heel, R. C., Brogden, R. N., Spreight, T. M., and Avery, G. S. Tamoxifen: A review of its pharmacological properties and therapeutic use in the treatment of breast cancer. *Drugs* 16: 1 (1978).

15. Buckley, M. M. T., and Goa, K. L. Tamoxifen: A reappraisal of its pharmacodynamic and pharmacokinetic properties, and therapeutic use. *Drugs* 37: 45 (1989).

16. Patterson, J. S. Nolvadex (tamoxifen) as an anti-cancer agent in humans. In *Non-steroid Antiestrogens,* D. J. A. Sutherland and V. C. Jordan, eds. Sydney: Academic Press, 1981, 143–163.

17. Scott, G. K., Kushner, P., Vigne, J. L., and Benz, C. C. Truncated forms of DNA-binding estrogen receptors in human breast cancer. *Amer. Soc. Clin. Invest.* 88: 700 (1991).

18. Fuqua, S. A. W., Fitzgerald, S. D., Chamness, G. C., Tandom, A. K., McDonnell, D. P., Nawaz, Z., and O'Malley, B. W. A variant human breast tumor estrogen receptor with constitutive transcriptional activity. *Cancer Res.* 51: 105 (1991).

19. Dickson, R. B., and Lippman, M. E. Estrogenic regulation of growth and polypeptide growth factor secretion in human breast carcinoma. *Endocrin. Rev.* 8: 29 (1987).

20. Touchette, N. Tamoxifen resistance in breast cancer. *JNIH Res.* 4: 67 (1992).

21. Miller, M. A., Lippman, M. E., and Katzenellenbogen, B. S.

Antiestrogen binding in antiestrogen growth resistant estrogen-responsive clonal variants of MCF-7 human breast cancer cells. *Cancer Res.* 44: 5038 (1984).

22. Preece, P. E., Wood, R. A. B., Mackie, C. R., and Cuschieri, A. Tamoxifen as initial sole treatment of localized breast cancer in elderly women: A pilot study. *Brit. Med. J.* 284: 869 (1982).

23. Stewart, H. J., Forrest, A. P. M., and Gunn, J. M. The tamoxifen trial—a double blind comparison with stilbestrol in postmenopausal women with advanced breast cancer. *Eur. J. Cancer* 1 (Supplement): 83 (1980).

24. Ingle, J. N., Ahmann, D. L., Green, S. J., Edmonson, J. H., Craegan, E. T., Hahn, R. G., and Rubin, J. Randomized clinical trial of diethylstilbestrol versus tamoxifen in postmenopausal women with advanced breast cancer. *N. Engl. J. Med.* 304: 16 (1981).

25. Heuson, J. C. Current overview of EORTC clinical trials with tamoxifen. *Cancer Treat. Rep.* 60: 1463 (1976).

26. Nemoto, T., Patel, J., Rosner, D., and Dao, T. L. Tamoxifen (Nolvadex) versus adrenalectomy in metastatic breast cancer. *Cancer* 53: 1333 (1984).

27. Kiang, D. T., Frenning, D. H., Vosika, G. J., and Kennedy, B. J. Comparison of tamoxifen and hypophysectomy in breast cancer treatment. *Cancer* 45: 1322 (1980).

28. Smith, I. E., Harris, A. L., Morgan, M., Gazet, J. C., and McKinna, J. A. Tamoxifen versus aminoglutethimide in advanced breast carcinoma: A randomized crossover trial. *Brit. Med. J.* 283: 1432 (1981).

29. Legha, S. S., Davis, H. L., and Muggia, F. M. Hormonal therapy of breast cancer: New approaches and concepts. *Ann. Intern. Med.* 88: 69 (1978).

30. Buchanan, R. B., Blamey, R. W., Durrant, K. R., Howell, A., Patterson, A. G., Preece, P. E., Smith, D. C., Williams, C. J., and Wilson, R. G. A randomized comparison of tamoxifen with surgical oophorectomy in premenopausal patients with advanced breast cancer. *J. Clin. Oncol.* 4: 1326 (1986).

31. Ingle, J. N., Krook, J. E., Green, S. J., Kubista, T. P., Everson, L. K., Ahmann, D. L., Chang, M. N., Bisel, H. F., Windschitl, H. E., Twito, D. F., and Pfeife, D. M. Randomized trial of bilateral oophorectomy versus tamoxifen in premenopausal women with metastatic breast cancer. *J. Clin. Oncol.* 4: 178 (1986).

32. Fornander, T., Rutqvist, L. E., Cedermark, B., Glas, V., Matts-

son, A., Silfversward, C., Skoog, L., Somell, A., Theve, T., Wilking, I., and Askergren, J. Adjuvant tamoxifen in early breast cancer: Occurrence of new primary cancers. *Lancet* 1: 117 (1989).

33. Anderson, M., Storm, H., and Mouridsen, H. T. Incidence of new primary cancers after adjuvant tamoxifen therapy and radiotherapy for early breast cancer. *J. Natl. Cancer. Inst.* 83: 1013 (1991).

34. DeMuylder, X., Neven, P., De Somer, M., Van Belle, Y., Vanderrick, G., and DeMuylder, E. Endometrial lesions in patients undergoing tamoxifen therapy. *Int. J. Gynecol. Obstet.* 36: 127 (1991).

35. Bush, T. L., and Helzlsouer, K. J. Tamoxifen for the primary prevention of breast cancer: A review and critique of the concept and trial. *Epidem. Rev.* 15: 233 (1993).

36. Jungi, F., and Wagen-Knecht, L. Tamoxifen alone or combined with multiple drug chemotherapy in disseminated breast carcinoma. *Proc. Amer. Assoc. Cancer Res. and Amer. Soc. Clin. Oncol.* 17: 312 (1977).

37. Lerner, H. J., Band, P. R., Israel, L., and Leung, B. S. Phase II study of tamoxifen: Report of 74 patients with stage IV breast cancer. *Cancer Treat. Rep.* 60: 1431 (1976).

38. Nevassaari, K., Heikkinein, M., and Taskinen, P. J. Tamoxifen and thrombosis. *Lancet* 2: 946 (1978).

39. Bratherton, D. G., Brown, C. H., Buchanan, R., Hall, V., Kingsley, E. N., and Pillers, E. M. A comparison of two doses of tamoxifen (Nolvadex) in postmenopausal women with advanced breast cancer: 10 mg bd versus 20 mg bd. *Brit. J. Cancer* 50: 199 (1984).

40. Ingle, J. N., Twito, D. I., Schaid, D. J., Colliman, S. A., and Krook, J. E. Randomized clinical trial of tamoxifen alone or combined with fluoxymesterone in postmenopausal women with metastatic breast cancer. *J. Clin. Oncol.* 6: 825 (1988).

41. Cocconi, D., DeLisi, V., Boni, C., Mori, P., and Malacarne, P. Chemotherapy versus combination of chemotherapy and endocrine therapy in advanced breast cancer: A prospective randomized study. *Cancer* 51: 581 (1983).

42. Gasparini, G., Canobbio, L., Galligioni, E., Fassio, T., and Brema, F. Sequential combination of tamoxifen and high dose medroxyprogesterone acetate: Therapeutic and endocrine effects in post-menopausal advanced breast cancer patients. *Eur. J. Cancer Clin. Oncol.* 23: 1451 (1987).

43. Margreiter, R., and Wiegele, J. Tamoxifen (Nolvadex) for premenopausal patients with advanced breast cancer. *Breast Cancer Res. Treat.* 4: 45 (1984).

44. Plotkin, D., Lechner, J. J., Jung, W. E., and Rosen, P. J. Tamoxifen flare in advanced breast cancer. *J. Amer. Med. Assoc.* 240: 2644 (1978).

45. Glick, J. H., Creech, R. H., Torri, S., Holroyde, C., and Brodovsky, H. Randomized clinical trial of tamoxifen plus sequential CMF chemotherapy versus tamoxifen alone in postmenopausal women with advanced breast cancer. *Breast Cancer Res. Treat.* 1: 59 (1981).

46. O'Connell, T. X. Hypercalcemia induced by tamoxifen. *Amer. J. Surg.* 141: 277 (1981).

47. Fisher, B., Costantino, J., Redmond, C., Poisson, R., Bowman, D., Couture, J., Dimitrov, N. V., Wolkmark, N., Wickerman, L., Fisher, E., et al. A randomized clinical trial evaluating tamoxifen in the treatment of patients with node-negative breast cancer who have estrogen-receptor positive tumors. *N. Engl. J. Med.* 320: 479 (1989).

48. Nayfield, S. G., Karp, J. E., Ford, L. G., Dorr, F. A., and Kramer, B. S. Potential role of tamoxifen in prevention of breast cancer. *J. Natl. Cancer Inst.* 83: 1450 (1991).

49. Ching, C. K., Smith, P. G., and Long, R. G. Tamoxifen-associated hepatocellular damage and agranulocytosis. *Lancet* 2: 940 (1992).

50. Gal, D., Kopel, S., Bashevkin, M., Lebowitcz, L., Lev, R., and Tancer, M. L. Oncologic potential of tamoxifen on endometria of postmenopausal women with breast cancer—preliminary report. *Gynecol. Oncol.* 42: 120 (1991).

51. Malfetano, J. H. Tamoxifen-associated endometrial carcinoma in postmenopausal breast cancer patients. *Gynecol. Oncol.* 39: 82 (1990).

52. Magriples, J., Naftolin, F., Schwartz, P. E., and Carcangiu, M. L. High-grade endometrial carcinoma in tamoxifen-treated breast cancer patients. *J. Clin. Oncol.* 11: 485 (1993).

53. Kaiser-Kupfer, M. I., and Lippmann, M. E. Tamoxifen retinopathy. *Cancer Treat. Rep.* 62: 315 (1978).

54. Pavlidis, N. A., Petris, C., Briassoulis, E., and Klouvas, G. Clear evidence that long-term, low-dose tamoxifen treatment can induce ocular toxicity. *Cancer* 69: 2961 (1992).

55. Gerlach, J. H., Kartner, N., Bell, D. R., and Ling, V. Multidrug resistance. *Cancer Surv.* 5: 25 (1986).

56. Pastan, I., and Gottesman, M. Multi-drug resistance in human cancer. *N. Engl. J. Med.* 316: 1388 (1987).

57. Shutt, D. A. The effects of plant estrogens on animal reproduction. *Endeavour* 35: 110 (1976).

58. Setchell, K. D. R., Borriello, S. P., Hulme, P., Kirk, D. N., and Axelson, M. Nonsteroidal estrogens of dietary origin: Possible roles in hormone-dependent disease. *Amer. J. Clin. Nutr.* 40: 569 (1984).

59. Jordan, V. C., Robinson, S. P., and Welshons, W. W. Resistance to antiestrogen therapy. In *Drug Resistance,* D. Kessle, ed. Boca Raton, Fla.: CRC Press, 1987, 403–427.

60. Osborne, C. K., Coronado, E., Allred, D. C., Wiebe, V., and DeGregorio, M. Acquired tamoxifen resistance correlated with reduced breast tumor levels of tamoxifen and isomerization of trans-4-hydroxytamoxifen. *J. Natl. Cancer Inst.* 83: 1477 (1991).

61. Colletta, A. A., Wakefield, L. M., Howell, F. V., Van Roozendal, K. E. P., Danielpour, D., Ebb, S. R., Spoun, M. B., and Baum, M. Antiestrogens induce the secretion of active transforming growth factors beta from human fetal fibroblasts. *Brit. J. Cancer.* 62: 405 (1990).

62. Osborne, C. K., Coronado, E. B., and Robinson, J. P. Human breast cancer in the athymic nude mouse: Cytostatic effects of long-term antiestrogen therapy. *Eur. J. Cancer Clin. Oncol.* 23: 1189 (1987).

63. Osborne, C. K., Hobbs, K., and Clark, G. M. Effect of estrogens and antiestrogen on growth of human breast cancer cells in athymic nude mice. *Cancer Res.* 45: 584 (1985).

64. Taylor, S. G., Gelman, R. S., Falkson, G., and Cummings, F. J. Combination chemotherapy compared to tamoxifen as initial therapy for Stage IV breast cancer in elderly women. *Ann. Intern. Med.* 104: 455 (1986).

65. Pritchard, K. I., Thomson, D. B., Myers, R. E., Sutherland, D. J. A., Moggs, B. G., and Meakin, J. W. Tamoxifen therapy in premenopausal patients with metastatic breast cancer. *Cancer Treat. Rep.* 64: 787 (1980).

66. National Institutes of Health Consensus Development Conference Statement: Treatment of Early Stage Breast Cancer. National Institutes of Health, Bethesda, Md., June 18–21, 1990.

67. Rutqvist, L. E., Cedarmark, B., Glas, U., Johansson, H., Nordenskjold, B., Skoog, L., Sommell, A., Theve, T., Friberg, S., and Askergren, J. The Stockholm trial on adjuvant tamoxifen in early breast cancer. Correlation between estrogen receptor level and treatment effect. *Breast Cancer Res. Treat.* 10: 255 (1987).

68. Breast Cancer Trials Committee, Scottish Cancer Trials Office

(MRC). Adjuvant tamoxifen in the management of operable breast cancer: The Scottish trial. *Lancet* 2: 171 (1987).

69. CRC Adjuvant Breast Trial Working Party. Cyclophosphamide and tamoxifen as adjuvant therapies in the management of breast cancer. *Brit. J. Cancer* 57: 604 (1988).

70. Fisher, B., and Redmond, C. K. A clinical trial to determine the worth of tamoxifen for preventing breast cancer. National Surgical Adjuvant Breast and Bowel Project Group (NSABP) Protocol P-1, December 20, 1991. Unpublished.

71. Stone, R. NIH fends off critics of tamoxifen study. *Science* 258: 734 (1992).

72. Jordan, V. C. Overview from the international conference on long-term tamoxifen therapy for breast cancer. *J. Natl. Cancer Inst.* 84: 231 (1992).

73. Baum, M., Houghton, J., and Riley, D. Results of the cancer research campaign adjuvant trial for perioperative cyclophosphamide and long-term tamoxifen in early breast cancer reported at the tenth year follow-up. *Acta Oncol.* 31: 251 (1992).

74. Gerner, E. W. Ocular toxicity of tamoxifen. *Ann. Ophthalmol.* 21: 420 (1989).

75. Raloff, J. Tamoxifen quandary: Promising cancer drug may hide troubling dark side. *Sci. News* 141: 266 (1992).

76. Han, X., and Liehr, J. G. Induction of covalent DNA adducts in rodents by tamoxifen. *Cancer Res.* 52: 1360 (1992).

77. Coradini, D., Cappelletti, V., Granata, G., and Difronzo, G. Activity of tamoxifen and its metabolism on endocrine-dependent and endocrine-independent breast cancer cells. *Tumor Biol.* 12: 149 (1991).

78. Gottardis, M. M., Wagner, R. J., Borden, E. C., and Jordan, V. C. Differential ability of antiestrogens to stimulate breast cancer cells (MCF-7) growth in vivo and in vitro. *Cancer Res.* 49: 4765 (1989).

79. Fendl, K. C., and Zimniski, S. J. Role of tamoxifen in the induction of hormone-independent rat mammary tumors. *Cancer Res.* 52: 235 (1992).

80. Hoogstraten, B., Gad-El-Mawia, N., Maloney, T. R., Fletcher, W. S., Vaughn, C. B., Tranum, B. L., Athens, J. W., Costanzi, J. J., and Foulkes, M. Combined modality therapy for first recurrence of breast cancer. *Cancer* 54: 2248 (1984).

81. Jiang, S. Y., and Jordan, V. C. A molecular strategy to control tamoxifen resistant breast cancer. *Cancer Surv.* 14: 55 (1992).

82. DeGregorio, M. W. Is tamoxifen chemoprevention worth the risk in healthy women? *JNIH Res.* 4: 84 (1992).

83. Bush, T. L., Fried, L. P., and Barett-Connor, E. Cholesterol, lipoproteins and coronary heart disease in women. *Clin. Chem.* 34: B60 (1988).

84. Stampfer, Meir J., and Colditz, Graham A. Estrogen replacement therapy and coronary heart disease: A quantitative assessment of the epidemiologic evidence. *Prevent. Med.* 20: 47–63 (1991).

85. Rossner, S., and Wallgren, A. Serum lipoproteins and proteins after breast cancer surgery and effects of tamoxifen. *Atherosclerosis* 52: 339 (1984).

86. Bruning, P. E., Banfrer, J. M. G., Hart, A. A. M., deJorg-Bakker, M., Linders, D., VanLoor, J., and Nooyen, W. J. Tamoxifen serum lipoproteins and cardiovascular risk. *Brit. J. Cancer* 58: 497 (1988).

87. Noguchi, M., Taniya, T., Tajiri, K., Miwa, K., Miyazaki, I., Koshino, H., Mabuchi, H., and Nonomura, A. Fatal hyperlipidemia in a case of metastatic breast cancer treated by tamoxifen. *Brit. J. Surg.* 74: 586 (1987).

88. Love, R. R., Newcomb, P. A., Wiebe, D. A., Svrawicz, T. S., Jordan, V. C., Carbone, P. P., and Demets, D. C. Lipid and lipoprotein effects of tamoxifen therapy in postmenopausal patients with node-negative breast cancer. *J. Natl. Cancer Inst.* 83: 1327 (1990).

89. McDonald, C. C., and Stewart, H. J. Fatal myocardial infarction in the Scottish adjuvant tamoxifen trial. *Brit. Med. J.* 303: 435 (1991).

90. Ryan, W. G., Wolter, J., and Bagdade, J. D. Apparent beneficial effects of tamoxifen on bone mineral content in patients with breast cancer: Preliminary study. *Osteoporosis Int.* 2: 39 (1991).

91. Wakley, G. K., Baum, B. L., Hannon, K. S., Bell, N. A., and Turner, R. T. The effects of tamoxifen on the osteopenia induced by sciatic neurotomy in the rat: A histomorphometric study. *Calcif. Tissue Int.* 43: 883 (1988).

92. Turner, R. T., Wakely, G. K., Hannon, K. S., and Bell, N. H. Tamoxifen prevents the skeletal effects of ovarian hormone deficiency in rats. *J. Bone Miner. Res.* 2: 449 (1987).

93. Wolter, J., Ryan, W. G., Subbaiah, V., and Bagdale, J. D. Apparent beneficial effects of tamoxifen on serum lipoprotein subfactions and bone mineral content in patients with breast cancer. *Proc. Amer. Soc. Clin. Oncol.* 7: 10 (Abstract 34) (1988).

94. Turken, S., Siris, E., Seldin, D., Flaster, E., Hyman, G., and Lindsay, R. Effects of tamoxifen on spinal bone density in women with breast cancer. *J. Natl. Cancer Inst.* 81: 1086 (1989).

95. Love, R., Mazess, R. B., Barden, H. S., Epstein, S., Newcomb, P. A., Jordan, V. C., Carbone, P. P., and Demets, D. L. Effects of tamoxifen on bone mineral density in postmenopausal women with breast cancer. *N. Engl. J. Med.* 326: 852 (1992).

96. Raloff, J. Tamoxifen and informed dissent. *Sci. News* 142: 378 (1992).

97. Henderson, B. E., Ross, R. K., and Pike, M. C. Hormonal chemoprevention of cancer in women. *Science* 259: 633 (1993).

98. Spicer, D., Shoupe, D., and Pike, M. C. GnRH agonists as contraceptive agents: Predicted significantly reduced risk of breast cancer. *Contraception* 44: 289 (1991).

99. Lippmann, M. E. Potential contributions of breast cancer biology to management of breast cancer. *Adv. Oncol.* 8: 26 (1992).

100. Recker, R. R., Davies, M., Hinders, S. M., Heaney, R. P., Stegman, M. R., and Kimmel, D. B. Bone gain in young adult women. *J. Amer. Med. Assoc.* 268: 2403 (1992).

Index

Page references to tables are in italic.

Bleeding problems (*continued*)
plant, 25; of chemotherapy, 19; of tamoxifen, *46,* 47, 48, 50

Blood, 19, 48; spitting up of, 49. *See also* Bleeding problems, as side effect; Thromboembolic disease, as side effect

Bonadonna, G., 22

Bone(s): breast cancer in, 47, 53, 55; scans of, 4, 56. *See also* Bone fractures; Bone marrow

Bone fractures: from cancer, 53; predictions about, 71, 73, 75, 79, 80; prevention of, 84–85, 89; and tamoxifen, 62–63

Bone marrow: suppression of, 18, 19, 20, 48; transplantation of, 25–26

Brain cancer, 13, 53

Breast cancer: cure rates for, 1, 7, 10, 37, 53, 63; diagnosis of, 1–2; drug-resistant, 55–56; drugs used in treatment of, 15–26; fear of, 61–62, 83, 88; hormone-insensitive, viii, 6, 29, 31, 34, 35–36, *39, 41,* 42, 43, 54, 76, 87; hormone-sensitive, viii, 6, 27–32, 35–36, 37, *38, 40,* 42, 43, 54, 55, 57, 70, 76, 78, 87; incidence of, vii, 13, 63, 75; kinds of, 6; mortality from, *7, 23,* 63; patient's prognosis, 7; prevention of, 62–63, 84–89; previous occurrence of, as risk factor, *10,* 11, 74–76; risk factors for developing, *10,* 11–13, 64, 75, 88; signs of, 2; spread of, 50, 52–55; stages

of, *4–5,* 7, 8–11; surgery for, vii, viii, 6–11, 53, 54; during tamoxifen trial, 69–70, 73, 78; types of therapy for, vii–viii, 6. *See also* Cancer Information Service; Cell growth; Chemotherapy; Hormonal therapy; Radiation; Recurrence of cancer; Survival rate; Tamoxifen; Tumor(s)

Breast Cancer Detection Demonstration Project (BCDDP), 65

Breath, shortness of, 49

Burning at injection site, *19, 20, 21*

CAF treatment regimen, 22

Calcifications, 3

Cancer Information Service, 1

Cancer Research Campaign Breast Cancer Trials Group, 76

Cancers, secondary, 19, 20, *46,* 72. *See also* Breast cancer; Tumor(s); *names of specific cancers*

Cardiovascular disease. *See* Heart problems

CAV treatment regimen, 22

Cell growth: and cytotoxic drugs, 15, 17, 18–19; and estrogen, 12; and hormone therapy, 15, 29–30, 59, 69, 77–78; as risk factor in recurrence, 42. *See also* Growth factors; S-phase, in breast cancer

Chemotherapy: amount of, 24–25; as breast cancer therapy, vii, viii–ix, 1, 6, 14–15, *23,*

High-density lipoprotein (HDL), 79

Hormonal therapy: for breast cancer prevention, viii, ix, 61–83, 85–86; as breast cancer therapy, vii, 6, 14, 33–44, 55; differences between chemotherapy and, 15–16; ideal patients for, 36–37; length of time in, 15, 43, 61, 76–77; resistance to, 55, 57–60, 78; tamoxifen compared to other kinds of, 35, 57. *See also* DES; Halotestin; Tamoxifen

Hot flashes, 46, 72, 73

Hypercalcemia, 47

Imperial Chemical Industries (Great Britain), 28

Indraductal carcinoma in situ (DCIS). *See* In situ breast cancer

Infection, 19, 25

Infiltrating breast cancer, 6, 42

In situ breast cancer, 6, 42, 64, 67, 69

Irritability, *46*, 47

Italy, tamoxifen trials in, 76

Kidney problems, 19, 20, 25

LCIS (lobular carcinoma in situ). *See* In situ breast cancer

LDL (low-density lipoprotein), 79–80

Leukemia, 13, 25

Leuprolide, 55

Liver problems: and breast cancer, 53; tests for, 4. *See also* Liver problems, as side effect

Liver problems, as side effect: of bone marrow transplant, 25; of chemotherapy, 19; of tamoxifen, *46*, 49–50, 77

Lobular carcinoma in situ (LCIS). *See* In situ breast cancer

Low-density lipoprotein (LDL), 79–80

Lump(s), 2–3

Lumpectomy, 7–11, 52

Lung problems: and breast cancer, 53; and chemotherapy, 19, 20

Lymph nodes: and chemotherapy, 37, 42; and spread of breast cancer, 4, 7–10, 22, 26, 53, 54

Lymphoma, 25

Mammogram, 2, 3, 6, 65, 84; accuracy of, 88–89; as risk factor, 12

Mastectomy, 7–11, 52, 53, 84, 88

Megestrol, 55

Melphalan, *16*, 20

Menopause: late, as risk factor, *10*, 11, 12; symptoms of, as tamoxifen side effect, 46–47

Menstruation: early, as risk factor, *10*, 11, 12, 64; irregularities in, and chemotherapy, 20, and tamoxifen, 46, 47, 72, 73

Metastatic cancer, 52–55; hormone therapy in, 33, 34, 43–44. *See also* Recurrence of cancer

Methotrexate, *16*, 18, 20, 21, 22, 54, 55

Mexate (Methotrexate), *16,* 18, 20, 21, 22, 54, 55, 56–57
Mitomycin, *16,* 20
Monoclonal antibodies, 87
Mouth sores, 19, 20
Mutamycin (Mitomycin), *16,* 20

Nail problems, 20
National Cancer Institute, 18, 62, 82
National Institutes of Health, 62
National Surgical Adjuvant Breast and Bowel Project (NSABP), 62, 63, 74
Nausea, as side effect: of chemotherapy, 18, 19, 20; of tamoxifen, *46,* 47
Needle biopsy, 3
Nerve damage, 21
Nervousness, *46*
Neurologic problems, 19, 21, 25
Nipples, 2
Nodes. *See* Lymph nodes
NSABP (National Surgical Adjuvant Breast and Bowel Project), 62, 63, 74

Obesity, *10. See also* Diet
Oncovin (Vincristine), *16,* 17, 21, 22
Osteoporosis. *See* Bone fractures
Ovaries: cancer of, 85–86; irradiation of, 33; removal of, 12, 29–30, 36–37

Pain: in arm, 49; in bone, 53; in breasts, 2, 3; in chest, 49; in leg, 49; and nerve damage from chemotherapy, 21
Palliative therapy, 53

Pathologist, 3, 6, *7,* 30, 42, 53–54
Payne, Donald M., 82
Perimenopause, 33–34
Pesticides, 13. *See also* Environmental pollution
Phenylalanine mustard (Melphalan), *16,* 20
Phlebitis, 48, *49,* 73
Phytoestrogens, 57
Platelets, 19, 48
Platinol (Cisplatin), *16, 19*
Platinum (Cisplatin), *16, 19*
Postmenopause: and combination chemotherapy, 22, *23,* 37; diet in, 84–85; and estrogen replacement therapy, 79–80, 85; and tamoxifen in breast cancer cases, viii, *23,* 27, 33–37, 42, 62, 74, 76, 82; and tamoxifen side effects, 46; and tamoxifen trial, 75, 76; treatment trends for breast cancer cases in, *40–41*
Prednisone, 22
Pregnancy, in tamoxifen trial, 70. *See also* Age: at birth of first child
Premenopause: and combination chemotherapy, 22, *23,* 36–37; hormonal therapy in breast cancer cases, viii, *23,* 29, 33, 36–37, 82; irradiation of ovaries in, 33; prevention efforts during, 85–86; risk factors associated with, 11; and tamoxifen in breast cancer cases, viii, *23,* 29, 36–37, 82; and tamoxifen side effects, 46, 82; and tamoxifen

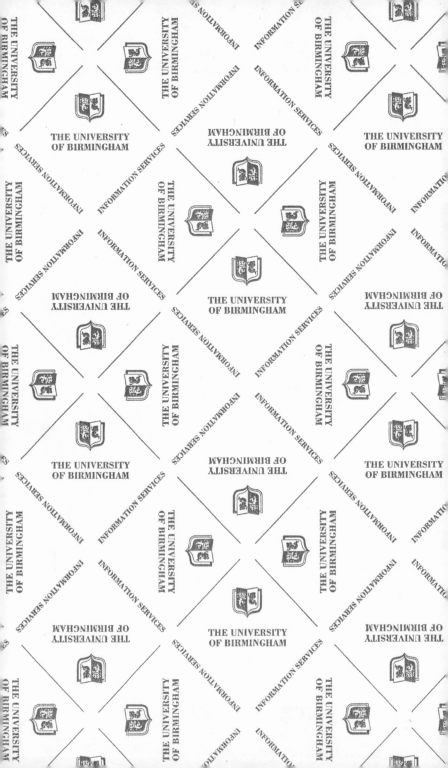